Microneedling in Clinical Practice

Microneedling in Clinical Practice

Edited by

Boris Stoeber, PEng, PhD
Faculty of Applied Science, University of British Columbia, Vancouver

Raja K Sivamani, MD, MS (Bioengineering), AP
Department of Dermatology, University of California at Davis
Department of Biological Sciences, California State University, Sacramento
College of Medicine, California Northstate University
Pacific Skin Institute
Zen Dermatology

Howard I. Maibach, MD
School of Medicine, University of California at San Francisco

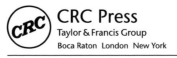

CRC Press
Taylor & Francis Group
Boca Raton London New York

CRC Press is an imprint of the
Taylor & Francis Group, an **informa** business

First edition published 2021
by CRC Press
6000 Broken Sound Parkway NW, Suite 300, Boca Raton, FL 33487-2742

and by CRC Press
2 Park Square, Milton Park, Abingdon, Oxon, OX14 4RN

© 2021 Taylor & Francis Group, LLC

CRC Press is an imprint of Taylor & Francis Group, LLC

Library of Congress Cataloging-in-Publication Data

Cataloging-in-Publication Data are on file in the Library of Congress

---

ISBN: 978-1-138-63315-5 (hbk)

ISBN: 978-1-138-03569-0 (pbk)

ISBN: 978-1-315-26561-2 (ebk)

Typeset in Times LT Std
by Cenveo® Publisher Services

Contents

Contributors

Heather A.E. Benson
School of Pharmacy
Curtin Health Innovation Research Institute
Curtin University
Perth, Western Australia

Kourosh Beroukhim
Department of Dermatology
University of California, Davis
Sacramento, California

John Havens Cary
Louisiana State University School of Medicine
New Orleans, Louisiana

Ashley Clarke
Department of Dermatology
University of Pennsylvania Perelman School of
    Medicine
Philadelphia, Pennsylvania

Michael L. Crichton
Heriot-Watt University
School of Engineering and Physical Sciences
    (EPS)
Edinburgh, United Kingdom

Institute of Mechanical, Process and Energy
    Engineering (IMPEE)
Edinburgh, United Kingdom

The University of Queensland
Delivery of Drugs and Genes Group
Australia

Australian Institute for Bioengineering and
    Nanotechnology (AIBN)
St. Lucia, Australia

ARC Centre of Excellence in Convergent
    Bio-Nano Science and Technology
The University of Queensland
Australia

Urs O. Häfeli
Faculty of Pharmaceutical Sciences
University of British Columbia
Vancouver, British Columbia, Canada

Yeakuty Jhanker
School of Pharmacy
Curtin Health Innovation Research Institute
Curtin University
Perth, Western Australia

Sahitya Katikaneni
Zosano Pharma
Fremont, California

Mark Kendall
The University of Queensland
Delivery of Drugs and Genes Group
Australia

Australian Institute for Bioengineering and
    Nanotechnology (AIBN)
St. Lucia, Australia

ARC Centre of Excellence in Convergent
    Bio-Nano Science and Technology
The University of Queensland
Australia

The University of Queensland
Diamantina Institute
Princess Alexandra Hospital
St Lucia, Queensland, Australia

The University of Queensland
Faculty of Medicine and Biomedical Sciences
Royal Brisbane and Women's Hospital
Herston, Queensland, Australia

Emrullah Korkmaz
Department of Mechanical Engineering
Carnegie Mellon University
Pittsburgh, Pennsylvania

JiYong Lee
School of Mechanical Engineering
Yonsei University
Seoul, South Korea

KangJu Lee
School of Mechanical Engineering
Yonsei University
Seoul, South Korea

Becky S. Li
Howard University College of Medicine
Washington, DC

Howard I. Maibach
Department of Dermatology
University of California
School of Medicine
San Francisco, California

Iman Mansoor
Department of Electrical and Computer
    Engineering
The University of British Columbia
Vancouver, British Columbia, Canada

O. Burak Ozdoganlar
Department of Mechanical Engineering
Carnegie Mellon University
Pittsburgh, Pennsylvania

Department of Materials Science and Engineering
Carnegie Mellon University
Pittsburgh, Pennsylvania

Department of Biomedical Engineering
Carnegie Mellon University
Pittsburgh, Pennsylvania

SeungHyun Park
School of Mechanical Engineering
Yonsei University
Seoul, South Korea

Aunna Pourang
Department of Dermatology
University of California, Davis
Sacramento, California

Tarl W. Prow
Biomaterials Engineering and Nanomedicine
    Strand
Future Industries Institute
University of South Australia
Adelaide, South Australia

Sahan A. Ranamukhaarachchi
Department of Electrical and Computer
    Engineering
University of British Columbia
Vancouver, British Columbia, Canada

WonHyoung Ryu
School of Mechanical Engineering
Yonsei University
Seoul, South Korea

Raja Sivamani
Department of Dermatology
University of California at Davis

Department of Biological Sciences
California State University
Sacramento College of Medicine
California Northstate University

Pacific Skin Institute
Zen Dermatology

Boris Stoeber
University of British Columbia
Vancouver, British Columbia, Canada

Janet Tamada
Scientia Bioengineering Consulting
Stanford, California

James H.N. Tran
School of Pharmacy
Curtin Health Innovation Research Institute
Curtin University
Perth, Western Australia

Samantha Tran
Stryker School of Medicine
Western Michigan University
Kalamazoo, Michigan

1

Microneedles and Transdermal Transport

Ashley Clark
University of Pennsylvania Perelman School of Medicine

Raja Sivamani
University of California-Davis
Pacific Skin Institute

1.1 Anatomy of the Skin

As the outermost layer of the body, the skin serves many roles including protection against UV radiation and microbes, regulating the movement of substances into and out of the body, and maintaining water and temperature equilibrium.[1] In order to perform its specialized functions, skin is divided into three layers: the epidermis, the dermis, and the hypodermis.

1.1.1 Stratum Corneum and Epidermis

The epidermis is the outermost layer of the skin and can range from 0.04 mm to 1.5 mm in thickness (Table 1.1), based on age, gender, ethnicity, and location on the body.[2] It is composed of self-regenerating stratified squamous epithelium, and serves as a protective barrier to the structures underneath. It is further separated into four layers: stratum corneum, stratum granulosum, stratum spinosum, and stratum germinativum. The stratum corneum consists of dead keratinocytes that form a relatively impermeable barrier to transdermal movement.

1.1.2 Dermis

The dermis is the layer of skin underlying the epidermis, measuring 1–2 mm in thickness.[6] It consists of nerves, vasculature, hair follicles, and glandular structures, held in place by a network of elastin and collagen fibers embedded in ground substance, which is the gel-like extracellular matrix that exists in the extracellular spaces.

1.1.3 Hypodermis

The hypodermis, also called the subcutaneous layer, is composed of approximately 3 mm of loose, well-vascularized connective tissue, and serves as adhesion to the bone and muscle. It also provides additional cushion and insulation.[6]

1.2 Modes of Transdermal Delivery

The skin is an appealing target for drug delivery for several reasons. Drug delivery through the skin is often minimally invasive and allows for more frequent administration. It also provides a larger surface area for drug absorption. And finally, transdermal drug delivery bypasses hepatic first-pass metabolism and deactivation through gastric enzymes.[7]

TABLE 1.1

Epidermal Thickness at Various Anatomical Sites

Body Site	Stratum Corneum (μm)	Mean Epidermal Thickness (μm)
Temple	6.3	61.4
Chest	6.5–12.8	56.0
Abdomen	6.3	61.3
Outer forearm	10.9–19.5	60.3
Leg	20.5–22.5	61.8
Dorsum of hand	9.3	84.5
Fingertip	160–209 (palm)	369.0

Adapted from Whitton et al.,[3] Robertson et al.,[4] and Bohlin et al.[5]

Unfortunately, the skin's effectiveness as a barrier makes transdermal drug delivery a difficult task. The stratum corneum is the primary gatekeeper, preventing the movement of large, polar substances across the skin. For this reason, a certain amount of creativity is required to purposely bypass the stratum corneum and deliver drugs directly to the vascular dermis.

Multiple solutions have been attempted to assist in drug delivery across the skin by increasing the permeability of the stratum corneum. These typically fall into two categories: chemical and physical enhancers (Table 1.2).

1. Chemical enhancers: Chemical enhancers work by interacting with the lipid bilayer of the stratum corneum to reversibly compromise the skin barrier, and allow for the penetration of drugs that would normally have difficulty crossing the stratum corneum. Although they are minimally invasive, chemical enhancers can cause significant irritation.[8] Listed below are various types of chemical enhancers.[9]
   a. Solvents (methanol, chloroform, acetone, pyrrolidones, sulphoxides)[10]
   b. Detergents
   c. Liposomes
   d. Nanoparticles
2. Physical Enhancers:[8]
   a. Iontophoresis: Iontophoresis involves the use of a small electrical current, either directly or indirectly, to aid in the movement of charged particles across the skin.
   b. Electroporation: Electroporation, unlike iontophoresis, uses high-voltage pulses to create small pathways within the skin's lipid bilayer, resulting in increased skin permeability.[11]

TABLE 1.2

Transdermal Drug Delivery Methods

Method	Mechanism	Examples
Chemical	Reversibly compromises the skin barrier when applied to the skin	Solvents Detergents Liposomes Nanoparticles
Physical	Current, ultrasound waves, and needles are used to create small holes in the skin	Iontophoresis Electroporation Sonophoresis Microneedles

c. Sonophoresis: Like electroporation, high-frequency sonophoresis also forms small holes in the skin to increase drug permeability. However, sonophoresis relies on ultrasound waves. It has been used to deliver topical steroids and NSAIDs.[12]

d. Microneedles: Microneedles form small holes in the stratum corneum, allowing for drug penetration through the least permeable layer of the skin. This method will be discussed in further detail below.

1.3 Microneedles

Microneedles can be a single microscopic needle or an array of them measuring approximately a few hundred microns in diameter, and up to 2500 μm in length. The needle's small size allows it to painlessly penetrate the epidermis when it is shorter (typically < 700 μm in length), making it incredibly useful for cosmetic, diagnostic, and therapeutic purposes.[13,14] As stated earlier, microneedles are used to form small conduits in the stratum corneum, allowing topical drugs to efficiently surpass this minimally permeable barrier.

Microneedles come in many shapes and sizes, and have been fabricated from various materials, including silicon, metal, polymer, glass, and ceramic.[15] There are generally three forms of microneedles:[14,15]

1. **Solid microneedles** are made from silicon, polymers, water-soluble compounds (e.g., maltose), and metals (e.g., stainless steel, titanium). They can be either uncoated or coated with the drug of interest. Uncoated solid microneedles can be used to create small holes in the skin before the application of a topical drug, to allow for more effective drug penetration. The tips of the microneedles can also be coated with a drug, allowing deposit of the drug into the deeper layers of the skin.

2. **Dissolving microneedles** are made from water-soluble materials such as polymers and sugars, and can dissolve once embedded into the skin. They often contain drugs encapsulated within the needle, and function similarly to a coated solid microneedle.

3. **Hollow microneedles** are often fabricated from metals or silicon and come in a variety of shapes, including cylindrical, conical, rectangular, and pyramidal. There is an opening either at the tip or on the side allowing liquid to flow into the skin. They are often used with a syringe or an actuator, for better control of drug flow.

1.4 Microneedles for Transdermal Drug Delivery

The use of microneedles for transdermal delivery of drugs enables circumvention of the thick stratum corneum by creating small conduits in the stratum corneum, allowing deeper penetration of drugs. Microneedles have been used to deliver desmopressin,[16] insulin,[17] vaccines,[18,19] and more. Differences in the needle length, width, and number can affect efficacy in drug delivery.

1.4.1 Depth of Microneedle Penetration

The depth of the micropore left by a given microneedle is indicative of the extent of the increase in permeability. In one study, using an optical coherence tomography (OCT) system to measure microneedle skin penetration in vivo, a 10×10 arrangement of needles 280 μm in height was measured to penetrate an average depth of 179 ± 14 μm into the skin. However, the average epidermal thickness measured under each micropore was 64 ± 19 μm, indicating that a component of the epidermis is compressed, and that the microneedles penetrate, on average, 61% of the epidermis.[20]

Another study (Table 1.3) used microscopy to assess the depth of penetration of various needle lengths and found that the mean depth corresponded well for shorter needle lengths (up to 1000 μm), but less well for longer needles (> 1500 μm).[21]

TABLE 1.3

Depth of Tissue Penetration of Various Needle Lengths

Needle Length (μm)	Mean Depth of Micro-Channels (μm ± SD)
250	235 ± 50
500	475 ± 35
1000	920 ± 75
1500	900 ± 500
2000	1275 ± 600
2500	1100 ± 650

Adapted from Sasaki et al.[20]

1.4.2 Rate of Micropore Closure

The rate of micropore closure is another important factor in determining its efficacy as a drug delivery mechanism. A slow closure rate provides adequate time for the drug to diffuse across the tissue. OCT imaging was used to assess changes in micropore depth over time. Again, using a 10 × 10 arrangement of 280 μm needles, the pore depth was measured to reduce from 158 ± 20 μm to 76 ± 13 μm, while the epidermal thickness under the micropore increased in thickness from 52 ± 11 μm to 92 ± 11 μm over a span of 85 minutes.[20] This increase might represent the intrinsic elasticity of the tissue, a regenerative process, or, most likely, a combination of both.

Various factors can slow resealing time, including increased microneedle length, number, and cross-sectional area, and application of an occlusive barrier (Table 1.4). In fact, one study found that doubling the length of the microneedle alone (from 750 μm to 1500 μm) can increase the skin resealing time by up to sixfold.[22] However, they also found that increasing the microneedle length, but not the number or cross-sectional area, resulted in increased pain. The study demonstrated that treatment with microneedles can increase skin permeability from 2 to 40 hours, depending on the geometry of the needle and the application of an occlusive barrier. Factors such as microneedle number, width (the size of the needle's opening), length, and spacing density can be adjusted to facilitate drug delivery without unnecessary pain.

1.5 Transdermal Extraction from the Skin

There has also been growing interest in the use of microneedles to painlessly sample from the interstitial fluid. Ideally, a high-density array of silicon-based hollow microneedles would remain in contact

TABLE 1.4

Microneedle Geometry and Corresponding Resealing Time

Treatment	Length (*l*) μm	Thickness (*t*) μm	Width (*w*) μm	Number of Microneedles	Skin Resealing Time in Minutes (Occluded)	Skin Resealing Time in Hours (Non-occluded)
A	750	75	200	50	30	2
B	750	75	200	10	3	2
C	500	75	200	50	22	2
D	1500	75	200	10	18	2
E	750	125	500	50	40	2
F	Hypodermic needle (26 gauge)				N/A	2

Adapted from Gupta et al.[22]

with the skin, allowing for continuous monitoring of the targeted substance.[23] The microneedle should be short enough to avoid penetration into the neurovascular-rich dermis and minimize pain and bleeding.[24]

Currently, the focus is on integrating microneedle arrays with sensors to allow for rapid analysis of the fluid sample. Engineering obstacles include needle mechanics to prevent clogging and buckling, as well as the creation of accurate micro-sensors.[23,25] Successful incorporation of microneedles into sensors would provide a noninvasive and painless method to measure drugs, electrolytes, and glucose levels, with minimal risk of infection.

While there are few clinical studies, early animal studies suggest that microneedle-based extraction may collect enough volume for biochemical analyses.[26] More clinical studies are needed to better evaluate small-volume sampling through microneedles.

1.6 Summary

The skin provides an efficient barrier against most compounds. However, its large surface area and its position as the outermost layer of the body make it a convenient and noninvasive location for drug delivery and interstitial fluid sampling. Microneedles, of various types, are a promising mechanism for both transdermal delivery and extraction due to their ability to traverse the mostly impermeable stratum corneum. Several factors, such as the needles' type and geometry, are important to keep in mind when developing and choosing microneedles, as they can influence the efficacy of drug delivery.

REFERENCES

1. Hussain SH, Limthongkul B, Humphreys TR. The biomechanical properties of the skin. *Dermatol Surg.* 2013;39(2):193–203.
2. June Robinson CWH, Siegel D, Fratila A, Bhatia A, Rohrer T. *Surgery of the Skin: Procedural Dermatology.* 3rd ed. London: Saunders; 2014.
3. Whitton JT, Everall JD. The thickness of the epidermis. *Br J Dermatol.* 1973;89(5):467–476.
4. Robertson K, Rees JL. Variation in epidermal morphology in human skin at different body sites as measured by reflectance confocal microscopy. *Acta Derm Venereol.* 2010;90(4):368–373.
5. Bohling A, Bielfeldt S, Himmelmann A, Keskin M, Wilhelm KP. Comparison of the stratum corneum thickness measured in vivo with confocal Raman spectroscopy and confocal reflectance microscopy. *Skin Res Technol.* 2014;20(1):50–57.
6. Washington N, Washington CW, Wilson Clive G. *Physiological Pharmaceutics: Barriers to Drug Absorption.* Boca Raton: CRC Press; 2000.
7. Escobar-Chavez JJ, Bonilla-Martinez D, Villegas-Gonzalez MA, Molina-Trinidad E, Casas-Alancaster N, Revilla-Vazquez AL. Microneedles: a valuable physical enhancer to increase transdermal drug delivery. *J Clin Pharmacol.* 2011;51(7):964–977.
8. Naik A, Kalia YN, Guy RH. Transdermal drug delivery: overcoming the skin's barrier function. *Pharm Sci Technolo Today.* 2000;3(9):318–326.
9. Jean L, Bolognia JVS, Cerroni L. *Dermatology.* 4th ed.: New York: Elsevier; 2018.
10. Lane ME. Skin penetration enhancers. *Int J Pharm.* 2013;447(1–2):12–21.
11. Brown MB, Martin GP, Jones SA, Akomeah FK. Dermal and transdermal drug delivery systems: current and future prospects. *Drug Deliv.* 2006;13(3):175–187.
12. Rodriguez-Devora JI, Ambure S, Shi ZD, Yuan Y, Sun W, Xui T. Physically facilitating drug-delivery systems. *Ther Deliv.* 2012;3(1):125–139.
13. Donnelly RF, Raj Singh TR, Woolfson AD. Microneedle-based drug delivery systems: microfabrication, drug delivery, and safety. *Drug Deliv.* 2010;17(4):187–207.
14. Bhatnagar S, Dave K, Venuganti VVK. Microneedles in the clinic. *J Control Release.* 2017;260:164–182.
15. Kim YC, Park JH, Prausnitz MR. Microneedles for drug and vaccine delivery. *Adv Drug Deliv Rev.* 2012;64(14):1547–1568.
16. Cormier M, Johnson B, Ameri M, et al. Transdermal delivery of desmopressin using a coated microneedle array patch system. *J Control Release.* 2004;97(3):503–511.

17. Gupta J, Felner EI, Prausnitz MR. Minimally invasive insulin delivery in subjects with type 1 diabetes using hollow microneedles. *Diabetes Technol Ther.* 2009;11(6):329–337.
18. Gill HS, Söderholm J, Prausnitz MR, Sällberg M. Cutaneous vaccination using microneedles coated with hepatitis C DNA vaccine. *Gene Ther.* 2010;17(6):811–814.
19. Ding Z, Verbaan FJ, Bivas-Benita M, et al. Microneedle arrays for the transcutaneous immunization of diphtheria and influenza in BALB/c mice. *J Control Release.* 2009;136(1):71–78.
20. Enfield JG, O'Connell ML, Lawlor K, Jonathan E, O'Mahony C, Leahy MJ. In-vivo dynamic characterization of microneedle skin penetration using optical coherence tomography. *J Biomed Opt.* 2010;15(4):046001.
21. Sasaki GH. Micro-needling depth penetration, presence of pigment particles, and fluorescein-stained platelets: clinical usage for aesthetic concerns. *Aesthet Surg J.* 2016;37(1):71–83.
22. Gupta J, Gill HS, Andrews SN, Prausnitz MR. Kinetics of skin resealing after insertion of microneedles in human subjects. *J Control Release.* 2011;154(2):148–155.
23. Mukerjee EV, Collins SD, Isseroff RR, Smith RL. Microneedle array for transdermal biological fluid extraction and in situ analysis. *Sens Actuators A Phys.* 2004;114(2):267–275.
24. Bruen D, Delaney C, Florea L, Diamond D. Glucose sensing for diabetes monitoring: recent developments. *Sensors (Basel).* 2017;17(8): pii: E1866.
25. Caffarel-Salvador E, Brady AJ, Eltayib E, et al. Hydrogel-forming microneedle arrays allow detection of drugs and glucose in vivo: potential for use in diagnosis and therapeutic drug monitoring. *PLoS One.* 2015;10(12):e0145644.
26. Taylor RM, Miller PR, Ebrahimi P, Polsky R, Baca JT. Minimally-invasive, microneedle-array extraction of interstitial fluid for comprehensive biomedical applications: transcriptomics, proteomics, metabolomics, exosome research, and biomarker identification. *Lab Anim.* 2018;52(5):526–530.

2

Skin Perforation and Solid Microneedles

Michael L Crichton[1,2,3]**, Mark Kendall**[2,3,4,5]

[1] *Heriot-Watt University, School of Engineering and Physical Sciences (EPS), Institute of Mechanical, Process and Energy Engineering (IMPEE)*
[2] *The University of Queensland, Australian Institute for Bioengineering and Nanotechnology (AIBN)*
[3] *ARC Centre of Excellence in Convergent Bio-Nano Science and Technology, The University of Queensland*
[4] *The University of Queensland, Diamantina Institute, Princess Alexandra Hospital*
[5] *The University of Queensland, Faculty of Medicine and Biomedical Sciences, Royal Brisbane and Women's Hospital*

2.1 Overview/The Goals of Skin Delivery (from a Medical Device Engineering Perspective)

The ability to place drugs and vaccines into the skin relies on having simple, effective ways to breach its surface and deliver therein. Achieving this requires the tough outer skin layer, the stratum corneum (SC), to be punctured, and the drug deposited in either the viable epidermis (VE) or the dermis below (or both). However, breaching skin's surface on a micro scale presents a challenge not just in the puncturing but also in how to place the corresponding payload in the vicinity of the cells or vessels we wish to reach. This becomes important when a technology (e.g., microneedles) is employed whose precise application requires the ability to ensure every dose is the same. For biological systems (e.g., the human body), this can be a significant challenge due to the biological variability of human skin. Indeed, the age, weight, sex, and environmental history of individuals will result in differences that must be overcome with any new technology targeting this area (1). This chapter will discuss the challenges of the skin's material properties and one way to achieve this with microneedles: solid microneedles.

2.2 Skin as an Engineering Material

2.2.1 The Material Composition of Skin

When considering a site for drug or vaccine delivery, its material composition must be considered. For skin, this means considering the three main constituent layers—the SC, VE, and dermis—and evaluating their distinct material properties. These have been discussed in the previous chapter, but they are discussed here with particular reference to their material properties.

2.2.1.1 The Epidermis (Comprising the SC and VE)

The epidermis of the skin represents a cellular epithelial tissue layer which ranges from the basal layer of the VE, through a process of vertical differentiation, to the tough keratinized cellular layer of the SC. Through this process, the cells' transition from newly divided to progressively flattened lose their nucleus and then harden (keratinize), resulting in a gradient of stiffness that increases from the base to the surface (2). The process takes about 28 days in a human (14 from basal layer to the bottom of the SC and then 14 for desquamation) and ensures the constant regeneration of our skin (3). However, as the thin, tough SC sits atop a soft, flexible layer of cells, the skin can deflect significantly when a force is applied—a positive, natural way to limit wounding but a challenge for engineers looking to puncture the skin to reach precisely within.

Potential variabilities in the epidermis relate to the hydration and environmental exposure of the skin layers, as these can significantly change the ability of layers to deform or puncture. For example, Wu et al. (4) noted that when human SC was stretched in high humidity, the skin showed corneocytes sliding over each other prior to the skin breaking. This behavior was not observed at low humidity and the skin fractured at an earlier point as a result.

The plate-like structure of the SC also presents a challenge for puncture, as it enables surface flexibility which allows deflection, avoiding penetration. While this may not be a problem for large devices by which very high pressures can be introduced (such as a vaccine syringe), placing smaller doses of vaccine/drug at precise locations can be a challenge.

2.2.1.2 The Dermis

Below the epidermis sits the dermis—a rich mesh of collagen, blood capillaries, cells, hair/sebum follicles, and nerve endings, embedded in a proteoglycan and hyaluronic acid gel (5). This layer can be further split into the papillary dermis (the upper dermis around the base of the epidermis) and the reticular dermis (the lower dermis). The papillary dermis has a finer mesh of collagen than the reticular dermis and contains smaller capillary ends; the reticular dermis has larger collagen bundles forming its structure and large capillaries (6). This composition means that the tissue has a range of properties that can challenge the engineer looking to deliver drugs or vaccine within. The collagen fibers in particular give an overall structural strength to the skin that enables it to be flexible but hard to puncture.

2.2.2 The Scale Dependency of Skin

One of the challenges for the development of novel micron-scale devices such as microneedles has been limited material property knowledge of skin's layers. Until relatively recently, the primary material properties of skin available were those that had been identified at the large scale (millimeters and above). However, recent studies on the micro and nano scale have shown that the tissue behavior is quite different at these scales (7). Indeed, as skin is a highly complex composite material, the relative influences of different physiological features become more significant as the scale decreases. For example, the VE and dermis may be considered a homogenous structure at the scale of millimeters or above, but on a smaller scale this is not the case. At the sub-millimeter and micron scales, features such as individual corneocytes, skin topography, collagen bundles, or rete ridges will influence the measured material properties (8). We have previously observed this, for example, where collagen presence in the dermis resulted in a bimodal distribution of elastic modulus in microscale testing.

For full-thickness skin, the elastic modulus of skin has been reported to vary from the low kilopascal range on the millimeter scale (9) up to megapascals at the small micro scale (7). As microneedles span these scales (from individual needles to full arrays), the designer of an array must consider how the skin's material behavior will affect its ability to puncture skin and deliver drug/vaccines.

2.3 Skin Fracture and Puncture

2.3.1 Skin Fracture

The ability to inject into skin has been of interest for hundreds of years with early needles and syringes using quills and animal bladders for fluid injection (10). In modern use, the conventional needle and syringe is credited to Dr. Alexander Wood, a Scottish physician, and concurrently Charles Gabriel

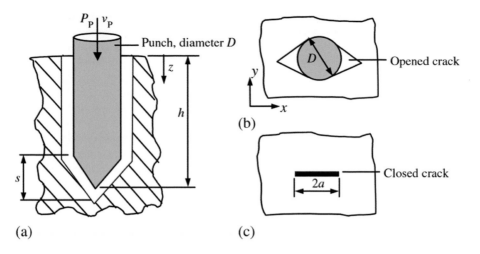

FIGURE 2.1 The mechanisms of puncture of skin as proposed by Shergold and Fleck (11), in which a sharp penetrator will expand a "crack" in skin to reach depth. (Reproduced with permission from ref. (11).)

Pravaz, a French orthopedic surgeon. Wood attached a graduated cylinder to a hypodermic syringe to deliver morphine into the veins of his patients, but there have been relatively few advances in the needle and syringe technology since then. One reason for this may be the complexity of puncturing skin in a minimally invasive way for fine positioning of a drug/vaccine payload.

The puncture of skin is a complex, multistage process in which a crack must be initiated to allow progressive entry into skin (Figure 2.1).

Specific aspects of the puncture process of skin relevant to microneedles include:

a. Contact and deflection phase:
   i. A sharp object contacts the skin either from directly above or at an angle.
   ii. The skin starts to deflect, with the SC distributing the force from the penetrator into and across the skin.
   iii. The stress (pressure) around the penetrator increases as deflection increases. While this is happening, the skin has deflected to the point where there is significant tension on the surface of the skin and the area of skin directly beneath the penetrator is being compressed (strain). The effect of this stress would be felt at a depth ten times the depth of the compression, reaching into the skin (12).

b. Puncture phase:
   i. As the tension on the SC increases and the compressive strain on the epidermis increases, a combined stress would eventually reach a critical point. This is where the surface fails and starts to rip/puncture. However, as the SC has a brick-and-mortar structure, this failure requires either delamination of corneocytes or ripping between them. When this event happens, the skin will dynamically puncture and the penetrator will progress into the skin.

c. Penetration phase:
   i. Beyond this initial puncture point, the progressive puncture of the skin requires the VE to continue to allow puncture—that is, to allow the penetrator to separate or burst the skin cells. At the same time, residual tension in the SC will provide friction against the penetrator to slow its entrance into the skin.
   ii. Pushing beyond the epidermis and into the dermis, the SC friction force continues, plus any force required for additional widening of the hole if the penetrator is not a uniform cylinder. Here, the collagen fiber mesh of the dermis is encountered. If the penetrator has

a very small diameter or sharp conical shape, it may be able to push between the collagen fibers, through the dermis. However, if it is of a larger scale, then it may encounter signifi-cant resistance at this point, requiring delamination or breakage of the collagen fibers to allow penetration.

These stages allow the progressive entrance of a penetrating object to the skin. Figure 2.2 shows a single microprojection from our work, penetrated into mouse skin tissue. Layer deflection and fracture are visible.

In studying the mechanisms of puncture, the engineering fracture toughness of a material becomes of interest. However, the orientation of testing is particularly important, as skin's high level of anisotropy (different properties in different testing orientations) results in differences in measured properties, as do differences in temperature or humidity. For example, in tensile testing of skin's SC, Koutroupi and Barbenel (13) measured a work to failure of 3.6 kJ/m^2, and a failure stress of ~60 MPa at around 75% humidity. However, Wildnauer et al. (14) found that skin failed at around 35 MPa, but with the failure strain ranging from 35% to 200% as relative humidity increased from 0% to 100%. From this, we can infer that there may be more challenges in getting microneedles to penetrate skin in high-humidity environments. This may be a consideration of importance for clinical use in many low-resource settings.

Other studies that have examined the cutting of full-thickness skin have shown lower fracture tough-ness values of around 2.5 kJ/m^2 in trouser tear testing (15). These values are however much lower than puncture toughness values that were presented by Davis et al. (16), with microneedle puncture giving around 30 kJ/m^2. This difference may be due to the increased complexity of the failure mode, in which skin has a vertical compressive behavior in addition to the tensile failure stresses present. So, while Shergold and Fleck suggest that soft solid penetration can be modeled as the opening of a crack, the actual initiation of this crack can absorb a lot of the applied energy. How this energy is absorbed was discussed by Yang et al. (17), who note that the skin has an impressive ability to adapt to high forces that would otherwise tear it.

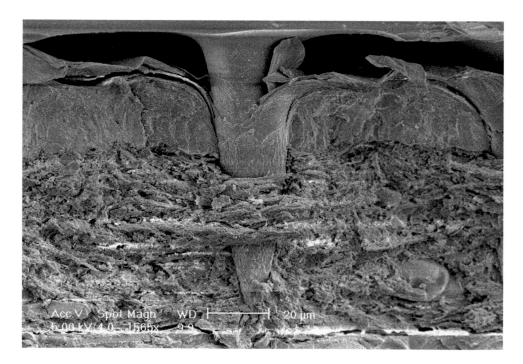

FIGURE 2.2   A nanopatch projection (original content) in mouse skin, following application at 2.3 m/s. This image was taken by freeze-fracturing skin with a nanopatch in place, showing the layers of skin (SC: stratum corneum; VE: viable epidermis) that have been deflected during the penetration process.

2.4 Microneedle Puncture of Skin

A range of designs of microneedles have been developed to place drugs and vaccines directly into precise locations in skin. These have the benefit of targeting skin layers that are otherwise difficult to reach and overcome the barrier properties of the SC. Solid microneedles have found widespread use in research and preclinical studies and are progressing in clinical studies. The concept of this microneedle approach is to have the simplest physical penetrator for the skin, with a drug/vaccine formulation that either dissolves from the surface once within the skin or can be applied after the perforation of skin by the microneedles. We will discuss microneedle perforation of skin in this chapter and coated microneedles in later chapters.

2.4.1 Microneedle Patch Manufacture

The manufacturing process of arrays of microneedles is dependent upon the materials to be used in the device, their strength, and the geometry of individual microneedles. Correspondingly, these then dictate how well the arrays puncture skin. Microneedle-manufacturing methods have been discussed in detail elsewhere (18, 19); we will briefly discuss some key approaches below.

a. Silicon manufacturing

Manufacturing from silicon makes use of either dry or wet etching of crystalline silicon wafers. This starts by defining a mask that is deposited on the surface, often using photolithography, which defines the areas for either anisotropic or isotropic etching. Wet etching is considered a simpler manufacturing process, as isotropic etching erodes material with orientation to the crystal structure of the material. This will give microneedle shapes that are generally blunter than dry etching (20). Dry etching, similar to that used in the microelectronic industry, can perform both anisotropic etching (etching vertically downward to make high aspect ratios) and isotropic etching (removal in all directions simultaneously). This approach can give some high-aspect-ratio structures with very sharp tips (sub-micron) (21, 22).

b. Metal manufacturing

Metal microneedles tend to either be based on the traditional needle and syringe, where multiple sharp tips are mounted upon a base, or make use of laser machining. Both methods have been used to create simple microneedle arrays. An example of the first is the manufacture of devices such as the "microneedle roller," now popular as a cosmetic device, with rows of sharp microneedles arranged on a roller to apply to the skin (23). Where laser-machined microneedles have been used, either a single row of microneedles has been created, or multiple rows have been machined and then bent to form the tips that will puncture the skin (24). This technique is again very good for producing very sharp tips.

c. Polymer manufacturing

Manufacture of polymer microneedles can be done using a variety of molding techniques in order to generate a range of microneedle profiles. These often require the manufacture of a "master" mold that can be manufactured from silicon, metal, or another polymer (e.g., PDMS/PMMA), into which the polymer can be formed (25, 26). Various forming techniques have been employed, which include direct injection molding, hot embossing, and melt-casting (discussed in more detail in ref. (27)). These processes enable arrays to be replicated at low cost and with fixed geometry.

While the manufacture method is unlikely in itself to indicate whether a clinical product will be achievable, some challenges affect manufacturing methods. For example, the cost of a single patch production and the ability to produce continuous production lines for millions of units per year will become important as such devices become standard in clinical use.

2.4.2 Microneedle Patch Application

Within the field of microneedles, there are significant challenges in getting arrays with large numbers of microneedles to puncture the skin. Some key points are:

a. High-density arrays—Skin is a topographically varied surface that can withstand large deformations prior to puncture. When there is a high-density array of microneedles (e.g., more than 500/cm²), a large number of discrete punctures must be created. This requires substantial energy. Naturally, as density and number of microneedles increase, the required force for skin puncture also increases. This can mean greater sensation for the patient and might require a larger/stronger device to be used for applications.

b. Tip sharpness—Varying the sharpness of the tips of microneedles can help control the puncture force. Increased tip sharpness not only reduces puncture force but also reduces the structural strength of the microneedles, leading to increased breakage risk. We have also observed that the capacity of the skin to distribute force from small penetrators (like microneedles) can limit the effectiveness of striving for progressively sharper tips, below the diameter of a few microns (28).

c. Bioactive component application—The location of the drug or vaccine payload is a significant consideration of microneedle design. If the payload is to be carried on the microneedle device, then the design must be adapted for this. For example, if this is a surface coating on the microneedles, the design will need to accommodate the extra surface geometries.

The application of microneedle patches to skin has been used with a variety of patch configurations, often with similar outcomes of the penetration force per microneedle. Roxhed et al. (29) applied a 25-microneedle array of sharp tip (<100 nm radius) microneedles to skin and measured penetration to require 10 mN per microneedle. Similarly, O'Mahony (30) found 15–20 mN per microneedle, and Resnik et al. (31) required around 15–30 mN per microneedle. These forces represent arrays of 10–100 microneedles, which give a total applicator force of 0.1–3 N. Although these forces are low, the need for consistent application may necessitate a controlled application approach/device.

Skin is a highly viscoelastic material, which means that any intention to puncture its surface will be dependent upon the velocity/strain rate at which puncture happens. If the device contacts slowly, a large deflection is likely, prior to puncture; if quickly, the deflection will be much lower. This has been observed when manual (hand) application of microneedle patches has been used for application. For example, Verbaan et al. (32) observed that with hand application of their patches, there was minimal increase in dye delivery into skin. However, when an applicator applied these at velocities of 1–3 m/s, flux increased by an order of magnitude above the manual application. We observed similar effects with penetration depth and patch surface area penetration doubled when dynamic application was used (33). An example of the differences observed by applying patches at difference velocities is shown in Figure 2.3. This data demonstrates one of the challenges in perforating skin with an array of microneedles: ensuring both that the penetration depth of microneedles is sufficient and that all the microneedles penetrate. As the energy of application decreases, some areas of the patch do not breach the surface (Figure 2.3).

These differences can be very important when using a device designed to reach into precise locations of the tissue.

2.4.3 Skin Substrate (Fat/Muscle)

The surface upon which the skin is sitting is one of the key determinants of where puncture will occur. Even with sharp penetrators, a soft layer underlying the skin may reduce penetration significantly, especially if there is fat/muscle variation. According to Meliga et al. (35), very sharp microneedles

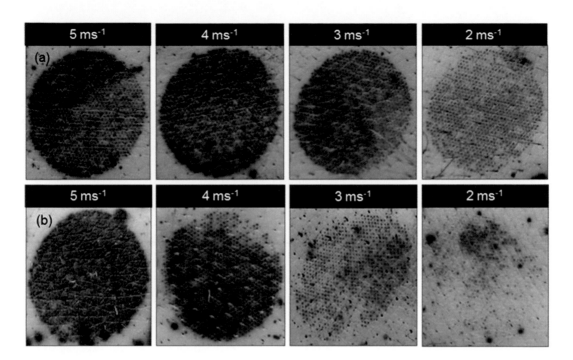

FIGURE 2.3 Delivery of dye when patches have been applied at increasing velocities. Lighter dye indicates lower delivered payload. These images are from arrays of 1316 microneedles of length 356 μm, spaced over a 15 mm radius. (a) is with a 36 g driving mass and (b) is using a 17 g driving mass (i.e., same velocity but half the mass). (Reproduced with permission from ref. (34).)

applied to mouse ear skin sitting on PDMS required almost 95% of the application energy to compress the soft substrate, compared to only 5% going to penetrate the mouse skin. While this is at the extreme ends of the comparison, it does allow us to speculate on how significant a clinical effect adipose tissue may introduce. The effect may be even more pronounced when a slow application is used and the skin has more time to deflect. In this situation, it is likely that the microneedles to be used will end up needing to be low-density arrays or have lengths that exceed 1 mm to ensure sufficient penetration. However, this may not be a problem: an ultrasound examination of skin layer thicknesses (36) observed that having microneedles of 1.5 mm length should ensure that the payload is always delivered into the dermis.

2.4.4 Microneedle Perforator/Enhancer Arrays

As discussed above, one of the simplest ways to use microneedles is to apply patches to the skin and then place a topical formulation on the surface. This then relies on diffusion into the pores created by the microneedle device to achieve the desired therapeutic outcome. This overcomes the ~500 Da cutoff for molecules passing through the surface of the skin (37), and as this is the key goal for this technology, the microneedles can be short. Correspondingly, this enables a low-pain, low-complexity approach.

The designs that have been employed for microneedle perforators or MEAs range in length, microneedle number, and shape. In general, these have numbers on the order of 100–1000 microneedles and are administered either by hand or with an applicator.

Microneedle length can be a strong determinant on their function. For example, Mikszta et al. (38) found that their 50-μm-long microneedles did not result in increased transdermal permeability, whereas 100-μm-long microneedlees increased permeability by 2800 times. This difference is most likely attributable to the ability of skin to deflect around short microneedles, but puncture with longer ones. In array form, Henry et al. (21) (using one of the earliest MEA designs) found that their 20×20 array of 150-μm-long, sharp-tipped (<1 μm) microneedles gave a permeability increase of up to 25,000 times. They observed that leaving the array in place longer (10 minutes–1 hour) resulted in a considerable increase in the permeability. This may be due to skin relaxing around the microneedles over time and the passage of the initial wound healing response.

The transport capability of skin once an MEA has been applied will depend upon the perforation depth of the tissue. If a drug is relatively small with high diffusion capacity, creating surface pores by microneedle application should be sufficient for therapeutic function. However, if rapid delivery to the bloodstream is a goal, it may be preferable to create pores that reach to the dermis where capillaries are located. This may be one reason for the very varied microneedle lengths that have been published to date. For example, in addition to the shorter microneedles discussed above, there have been many studies with long microneedles, such as that of Martanto et al. (24), which looked to increase insulin permeability into skin using 1000-μm-long microneedles.

To attempt to produce a more controlled-release approach to drug delivery once the pores were created, Pearton et al. used a hydrogel for delivery of plasmid DNA for gene regulation in the skin following application of 260-μm-long microneedles (4×4 array). Their 50–100 μm pores, combined with the hydrogel, allowed more precise gene regulation in the skin. These short conduits appear to be sufficient to improve drug delivery to a large extent. Wu et al. (39) observed similar-sized conduits by application of their 150-μm-long microneedles, giving 10^4- to-10^5-fold improvement in calcein.

The use of microneedle rollers has recently grown with a wide range of topical applications used. Enhancements in topical anesthetics (40), antiepileptic drugs (41), hair growth (42), and skin aging (43) have all been reported with the microneedle roller. However, even with very simple devices like these, there have been adverse clinical outcomes when used for cosmeceutical purposes. The rapid uptake of these devices by the cosmetics industry has resulted in some drugs approved for topical use only being introduced into the body. Clinical presentation with erythema and granulomas in the skin has been observed (discussed in ref. (44)). This is one problem with the perceived simplicity of these devices and the ease of obtaining them.

2.4.5 Challenges of MEAs

While MEAs have the potential to overcome the barrier properties of the SC, they rely on passive diffusion of the biological formulation into skin. This can make it difficult to deliver high doses, and a lot of the dose will be wasted on the surface of the skin.

The time of application and the inability to monitor dose delivery have made this technology less attractive for certain clinical applications. One example is in the area of vaccine delivery. Recent studies (e.g., ref. (45)) have noted that delivering vaccine directly to the epidermis and dermis in skin has the potential to generate immune responses with far less vaccine than traditional intramuscular injection. However, if only a small percentage of the applied dose reaches the skin, these benefits can be lost. And while this may not be a complete barrier to this technology, dose consistency is of great importance. For vaccines in particular, a threshold dose must be delivered to invoke immunity, which can be more difficult when relying on passive diffusion after microneedle application. However, for cheap compounds or drugs generally applied in topical form, the increase in dose that can enter the body will represent a significant advance.

2.4.6 Clinical Use

A key benefit of the solid MEA approach is that the clinical development of the microneedle device can progress independently of the drug or vaccine formulation. This might considerably simplify any regulatory process and might allow more rapid integration of the technology into the supply chain of particular drugs. However, it becomes important to ensure that the drugs to be used are suitable for internal delivery and not just as topical carriers.

2.5 Conclusions

Perforating skin on a micro scale remains a significant challenge for devices that aim to enable precision drug or vaccine delivery. Another complication is introduced when there is a large array of short microneedles, as this increases the risk of only partial surface puncture across the array. The result of these challenges is that an applicator of some type is often required to precisely position the microneedles where the drug should be deposited. Topical drug application to the site following surface puncture (or perforation) has the potential for simple, effective delivery of large-molecular-weight drugs and vaccines into the body. Although only a small amount of the molecule may actually reach its desired delivery location, the simplicity of the approach may reduce the regulatory challenges experienced by other, more complex formulation approaches.

REFERENCES

1. Diridollou S, Vabre V, Berson M, Vaillant L, Black D, Lagarde JM, et al. Skin ageing: changes of physical properties of human skin in vivo. Int J Cosmet Sci. 2001;23:353–62.
2. Kendall MAF, Chong Y-F, Cock A. The mechanical properties of the skin epidermis in relation to targeted gene and drug delivery. Biomaterials. 2007;28(33):4968–77.
3. Halprin KM. Epidermal "turnover time"—a re-examination. Br J Dermatol. 1972;86(1):14–9.
4. Wu KS, Dauskardt RH, van Osdol WW. Mechanical properties of human stratum corneum: effects of temperature, hydration, and chemical treatment. Biomaterials. 2006;27(5):785–95.
5. Juhlin L. Hyaluronan in skin. J Intern Med. 1997;242(1):61–6.
6. Sherman VR, Tang Y, Zhao S, Yang W, Meyers MA. Structural characterization and viscoelastic constitutive modeling of skin. Acta Biomater. 2017;53(Supplement C):460–9.
7. Crichton ML, Chen X, Huang H, Kendall MAF. Elastic modulus and viscoelastic properties of full thickness skin characterised at micro scales. Biomaterials. 2013;34(8):2087–97.
8. Crichton ML, Donose BC, Chen X, Raphael AP, Huang H, Kendall MA. The viscoelastic, hyperelastic and scale dependent behaviour of freshly excised individual skin layers. Biomaterials. 2011;32(20):4670–81.
9. Jachowicz J, McMullen R, Prettypaul D. Indentometric analysis of in vivo skin and comparison with artificial skin models. Skin Res Technol. 2007;13(3):299–309.
10. Norn S, Kruse PR, Kruse E. [On the history of injection]. Dansk Medicinhistorisk Arbog. 2006;34:104–13.
11. Shergold OA, Fleck NA, King TS. The penetration of a soft solid by a liquid jet, with application to the administration of a needle-free injection. J Biomech. 2006;39(14):2593–602.
12. Jung Y, Lawn B, Martyniuk M, Huang H, Hu X. Evaluation of elastic modulus and hardness of thin films by nanoindentation J Mater Res. 2004;19(10):5.
13. Koutroupi KS, Barbenel JC. Mechanical and failure behaviour of the stratum corneum. J Biomech. 1990;23(3):281–7.
14. Wildnauer RH, Bothwell JW, Douglass AB. Stratum corneum properties I. influence of relative humidity on normal and extracted human stratum corneum. J Investig Dermatol. 1971;56(1):72–8.
15. Shergold OA, Fleck NA. Experimental investigation into the deep penetration of soft solids by sharp and blunt punches, with application to the piercing of skin. J Biomech Eng. 2005;127(5):838–48.
16. Davis SP, Landis BJ, Adams ZH, Allen MG, Prausnitz MR. Insertion of microneedles into skin: measurement and prediction of insertion force and needle fracture force. J Biomech. 2004;37(8):1155–63.
17. Yang W, Sherman VR, Gludovatz B, Schaible E, Stewart P, Ritchie RO, et al. On the tear resistance of skin. Nat Commun. 2015;6:6649.
18. Donnelly RF, Raj Singh TR, Woolfson AD. Microneedle-based drug delivery systems: microfabrication, drug delivery, and safety. Drug Deliv. 2010;17(4):187–207.
19. Larrañeta E, Lutton REM, Woolfson AD, Donnelly RF. Microneedle arrays as transdermal and intradermal drug delivery systems: materials science, manufacture and commercial development. Mater Sci Eng R Rep. 2016;104(Supplement C):1–32.
20. Pearton M, Allender C, Brain K, Anstey A, Gateley C, Wilke N, et al. Gene delivery to the epidermal cells of human skin explants using microfabricated microneedles and hydrogel formulations. Pharm Res. 2008;25(2):407–16.

21. Henry S, McAllister DV, Allen MG, Prausnitz MR. Microfabricated microneedles: a novel approach to transdermal drug delivery. J Pharm Sci. 1998;87(8):922–5.

22. Jenkins D, Corrie S, Flaim C, Kendall M. High density and high aspect ratio solid micro-nanoprojection arrays for targeted skin vaccine delivery and specific antibody extraction. RSC Advances. 2012;2(8):3490–5.

23. Badran MM, Kuntsche J, Fahr A. Skin penetration enhancement by a microneedle device (Dermaroller®) in vitro: dependency on needle size and applied formulation. Eur J Pharm Sci. 2009;36(4–5):511–23.

24. Martanto W, Davis SP, Holiday NR, Wang J, Gill HS, Prausnitz MR. Transdermal delivery of insulin using microneedles in vivo. Pharm Res. 2004;21(6):947–52.

25. Moon SJ, Lee SS, Lee HS, Kwon TH. Fabrication of microneedle array using LIGA and hot embossing process. Microsyst Technol. 2005;11(4):311–8.

26. Manhee H, Dong-Hun H, Hyoun-Hyang P, Seung SL, Chang-Hyeon K, ChangGyou K. A novel fabrication process for out-of-plane microneedle sheets of biocompatible polymer. J Micromech Microeng. 2007;17(6):1184.

27. Tuan-Mahmood T-M, McCrudden MTC, Torrisi BM, McAlister E, Garland MJ, Singh TRR, et al. Microneedles for intradermal and transdermal delivery. EurJ Pharm Sci. 2013;50(5):623–37.

28. Crichton ML, Archer-Jones C, Meliga S, Edwards G, Martin D, Huang H, et al. Characterising the material properties at the interface between skin and a skin vaccination microprojection device. Acta Biomater. 2016;36:186–94.

29. Roxhed N, Gasser TC, Griss P, Holzapfel GA, Stemme G. Penetration-enhanced ultrasharp microneedles and prediction on skin interaction for efficient transdermal drug delivery. J Microelectromech Syst. 2007;16(6):1429–40.

30. O'Mahony C. Structural characterization and in-vivo reliability evaluation of silicon microneedles. Biomed Microdevices. 2014;16(3):333–43.

31. Resnik D, Možek M, Pečar B, Dolžan T, Janež A, Urbančič V, et al. Characterization of skin penetration efficacy by Au-coated Si microneedle array electrode. Sensors & Actuators A: Physical. 2015;232:299–309.

32. Verbaan FJ, Bal SM, van den Berg DJ, Dijksman JA, van Hecke M, Verpoorten H, et al. Improved piercing of microneedle arrays in dermatomed human skin by an impact insertion method. J Control Release. 2008;128(1):80–8.

33. Crichton ML, Ansaldo A, Chen X, Prow TW, Fernando GJ, Kendall MA. The effect of strain rate on the precision of penetration of short densely-packed microprojection array patches coated with vaccine. Biomaterials. 2010;31(16):4562–72.

34. Moronkeji K, Todd S, Dawidowska I, Akhtar R. In vitro quantification of optimal impact properties for microneedle penetration. In: Tekalur SA, Zavattieri P, Korach CS, editors. Mechanics of Biological Systems and Materials, Volume 6: *Proceedings of the 2015 Annual Conference on Experimental and Applied Mechanics*. Cham: Springer International Publishing; 2016. pp. 39–49.

35. Meliga SC, Coffey JW, Crichton ML, Flaim C, Veidt M, Kendall MAF. The hyperelastic and failure behaviors of skin in relation to the dynamic application of microscopic penetrators in a murine model. Acta Biomater. 2017;48:341–56.

36. Laurent A, Mistretta F, Bottigioli D, Dahel K, Goujon C, Nicolas Jean F, et al. Echographic measurement of skin thickness in adults by high frequency ultrasound to assess the appropriate microneedle length for intradermal delivery of vaccines. Vaccine. 2007;25(34):6423–30.

37. Bos JD, Meinardi MMHM. The 500 Dalton rule for the skin penetration of chemical compounds and drugs. Exp Dermatol. 2000;9(3):165–9.

38. Mikszta JA, Alarcon JB, Brittingham JM, Sutter DE, Pettis RJ, Harvey NG. Improved genetic immunization via micromechanical disruption of skin-barrier function and targeted epidermal delivery. Nat Med. 2002;8(4):415–9.

39. Wu Y, Qiu Y, Zhang S, Qin G, Gao Y. Microneedle-based drug delivery: studies on delivery parameters and biocompatibility. Biomed Microdevices. 2008;10(5):601–10.

40. Buhsem O, Aksoy A, Kececi Y, Sir E, Gungor M. Increasing topical anesthetic efficacy with microneedle application. J Cosmet Laser Ther. 2016;18(5):286–8.

41. Nguyen J, Ita KB, Morra MJ, Popova IE. The influence of solid microneedles on the transdermal delivery of selected antiepileptic drugs. Pharmaceutics. 2016;8(4):33.

42. Kim YS, Jeong KH, Kim JE, Woo YJ, Kim BJ, Kang H. Repeated microneedle stimulation induces enhanced hair growth in a murine model. Ann Dermatol. 2016;28(5):586–92.
43. Lee HJ, Lee EG, Kang S, Sung JH, Chung HM, Kim DH. Efficacy of microneedling plus human stem cell conditioned medium for skin rejuvenation: a randomized, controlled, blinded split-face study. Ann Dermatol. 2014;26(5):584–91.
44. Singh A, Yadav S. Microneedling: advances and widening horizons. Indian Dermatol Online J. 2016;7(4):244–54.
45. Fernando GJ, Chen X, Prow TW, Crichton ML, Fairmaid EJ, Roberts MS, et al. Potent immunity to low doses of influenza vaccine by probabilistic guided micro-targeted skin delivery in a mouse model. PLoS One. 2010;5(4):e10266.

3

Dissolvable and Coated Microneedle Arrays: Design, Fabrication, Materials and Administration Methods

Emrullah Korkmaz[1] and O. Burak Ozdoganlar[1,2,3]
[1] *Department of Mechanical Engineering, Carnegie Mellon University*
[2] *Department of Materials Sci. and Engineering, Carnegie Mellon University*
[3] *Department of Biomedical Engineering, Carnegie Mellon University*

3.1 Introduction

Delivering therapeutics and vaccines by cutaneous and transdermal routes offers unique advantages over prevailing oral and parenteral drug delivery methods [1, 2]. Transdermal systems deliver vaccines and therapeutics *through the skin* into the systemic circulation, whereas cutaneous systems deliver drugs *into the skin*, targeting certain skin microenvironments (e.g., epidermis and dermis). Both transdermal and cutaneous routes bypass the gastrointestinal (GI) tract, thereby improving bioavailability and potency of the delivered drugs, as well as reducing their side effects. Transdermal and cutaneous drug delivery routes also eliminate needle-stick injuries and needle reuse issues, and increase patient compliance since they cause little to no pain during administration. Moreover, these routes minimize or eliminate the need for, and the associated cost of, trained health care professionals for administration of drugs [1–4]. As a result, the number of transdermal and cutaneous drugs in the market and in the regulatory approval pipeline has been expanding significantly in the past few years [1].

Although many advantages of transdermal and cutaneous (i.e., intradermal) delivery have been well recognized, they have yet to be fully exploited. Transdermal and cutaneous routes present their own challenges: delivering drugs through these routes requires overcoming the physical barrier imposed by the stratum corneum (SC), the top layer of the skin [5]. Without a physical breach or chemical penetration enhancers, only small molecules (<500 Da molecular weight) can penetrate the SC [6–8]. This puts significant limits on the types of proteins, peptides, and genetic materials (i.e., polyplexes and recombinant viral vectors) that can be directly delivered to or through the skin, thereby hindering the use of transdermal and intradermal routes for a majority of vaccines and therapeutics without the use of specifically designed delivery systems [9, 10].

To mitigate the limitations associated with the transdermal and cutaneous delivery toward increasing the types of drugs that can be administered through these routes, as well as toward improving the delivery efficiency, microneedle array (MNA)-based trans/intradermal delivery systems have been developed in the past decade [2, 4, 11, 26]. These devices include an array of microneedles, each with dimensions ranging from 50 μm to 1 mm in width, and up to 1.5 mm in height. Microneedle arrays physically breach the SC layer and enable delivering therapeutics and vaccines to viable epidermis and dermis in a minimally invasive manner [1, 2]. Pioneering works have demonstrated that trans/intradermal delivery using MNAs can overcome the aforementioned challenges while retaining advantages of transdermal and cutaneous delivery [12–16, 26]. However, the full potential of MNA-based trans/intradermal drug delivery has not yet been realized, mainly due to considerable challenges in design, manufacturing, and administration of MNAs.

Currently, there are four major MNA-based trans/intradermal drug delivery concepts (Figure 3.1). The first concept is known as the *poke-and-patch* approach, where solid microneedles made of silicon, metals, or non-dissolvable polymers are used to precondition the skin by piercing the SC. The pores created

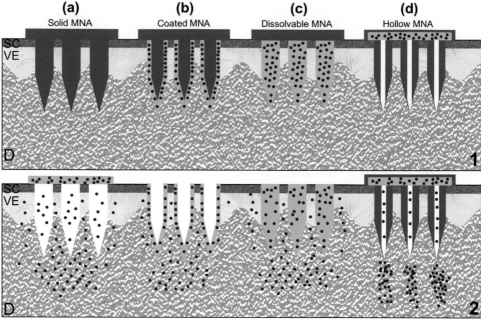

FIGURE 3.1 Microneedle-based trans/intradermal drug delivery concepts. **1. Types: (a)** Solid MNA, **(b)** Coated MNA, **(c)** Dissolvable MNA, and **(d)** Hollow MNA. **2. Methods: (a)** Solid microneedles are used to precondition the skin by piercing the stratum corneum to substantially increase the permeability prior to topical application of drug (*poke-and-patch*). **(b)** Drug-coated solid microneedles are inserted into the skin. Upon insertion of microneedles, the drug coating is dissolved into the skin, after which the microneedles are removed (*coat-and-poke*). **(c)** Dissolvable microneedles penetrate the skin, and then dissolve and deliver their cargo to targeted skin microenvironments *(poke-and-release)*. **(d)** Hollow microneedles are utilized to deliver liquid drug solutions into the skin *(poke-and-flow)*. SC: stratum corneum; VE: viable epidermis, D: dermis.

by the MNAs increase the permeability of skin to subsequent topical and transdermal-patch-based deliveries (Figure 3.1a) [6, 15–17]. However, since this method relies on passive diffusion of the bioactive cargo, it provides only limited spatial, dosage, and delivery rate control [6]. Furthermore, the MNA material should be carefully selected to prevent unwanted complications in the event of accidental breakage of the microneedles in the skin. Therefore, it is important to create these solid MNAs from biocompatible materials.

The second concept, the *coat-and-poke* approach, also uses solid microneedles created from silicon, metals, or non-dissolvable polymers. The microneedles are coated with the aqueous solution containing the drug to be delivered. Upon insertion, the drug coating is dissolved into the skin, after which the microneedles are removed (Figure 3.1b) [6, 18]. Although this method provides a better dosage and spatial control over the *poke-and-patch* approach, its capacity is limited to small quantities of drugs. Similarly to the *poke-and-patch* approach, the MNA materials should be carefully selected to avoid potential complications.

The third concept is the *poke-and-release* approach, in which MNAs are made from biodissolvable materials that encapsulate the drug within the microneedle material. Upon insertion into the skin, the MNAs dissolve rapidly and deliver their biocargo to targeted skin microenvironments. Dissolvable MNAs have been demonstrated to have sufficient strength to allow insertion, to dissolve within minutes in interstitial fluids of the skin, and to effectively release their biocargo [6, 19–21, 26, 67–68]. The dissolvable MNAs are made from biocompatible materials, and their full dissolution eliminates sharp or biohazardous waste (Figure 3.1c) [6, 19–21, 26, 69]. Therefore, dissolvable MNAs combine the physical toughness of solid microneedles with relatively high bioactive material capacity and controllable delivery rate, while possessing other desired attributes of simple and low-cost fabrication, storage, and application.

The last microneedle concept, the *poke-and-flow* approach, utilizes hollow microneedles attached to a reservoir of bioactive cargo [6, 22] (Figure 3.1d). The hollow microneedles and associated design, manufacturing, and administration aspects will be covered in Chapter 4.

This chapter focuses on design, manufacturing, and administration aspects of the MNAs for the *coat-and-poke* and *poke-and-release* concepts. The following section discusses the geometric design considerations for both the individual and the array of microneedles. Subsequently, we describe the prevailing fabrication methods for the MNAs. We then discuss the selection of MNA materials. Next, we discuss the administration methods, which is critical in realizing precise and reproducible delivery using MNAs.

3.2 Microneedle and Array Designs

Realizing the true potential of MNAs depends critically upon precise and effective delivery of their biocargo to targeted skin microenvironments in a minimally invasive manner [23–26]. The MNAs must penetrate the SC with minimum force and without mechanical failure to deliver their biocargo to the epidermis and/or dermis. Penetration and cargo delivery performance of MNAs are highly correlated with the geometry of individual microneedles and the array, MNA materials, the MNA administration method, and the skin-tissue characteristics [23]. Ideally, the microneedle design and administration method should maximize the number and portion of the microneedles that penetrate the skin with low insertion forces to achieve an optimal and precise delivery performance with minimum tissue damage. Further, clinically relevant microneedle and array designs should enable controllable and reproducible delivery location and dose. This section focuses on geometric aspects of microneedle and array designs, and discusses the critical design aspects for successful and reproducible penetration of MNAs into the skin with minimum tissue damage toward optimal biocargo delivery.

The geometric parameters of the microneedle and array designs (Figure 3.2) include tip radius, apex shape and dimensions, stem shape and dimensions, bevel angle, fillet radius at the base of the microneedles, tip-to-tip distance of microneedles in the array, and overall array size. These parameters directly impact the mechanical performance (i.e., penetration and failure characteristics) of MNAs, their biocargo capacity, cargo delivery location, and the tissue damage caused by the MNA insertion [23–26]. In general, the cutting and deformation of skin tissue arise from the thrust (axial) force at the microneedle tip and the friction force between the microneedle surface (including that of the stem) and the skin tissue.

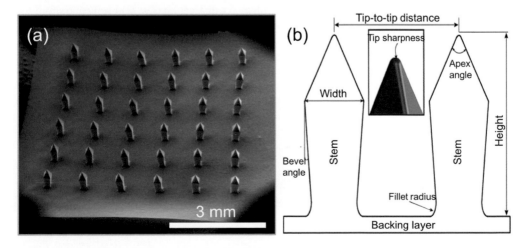

FIGURE 3.2 MNA design parameters: **(a)** A 6 × 6 MNA with negative bevel obelisk microneedles and with a total size of 8 mm × 8 mm. **(b)** Microneedle and array geometric parameters indicated on a negative bevel obelisk needle [24, 26].

Tip sharpness, quantified by *the tip radius*, is a critical factor for skin penetration. Sharper microneedles can penetrate the skin with low insertion forces [6, 23, 26]. *Apex shape and dimensions* control the force distribution during penetration and deeper tissue insertion. Symmetric apex geometries and smooth edges can provide more uniform force distributions, thereby reducing the possibility of microneedle failure during insertion. Microneedles with smaller apex angles lead to lower penetration forces. *Stem shape and dimensions* not only affect the insertion forces but also dictate the delivery location and depth. Shorter microneedles (<300 μm in height) may not penetrate the skin at low application force and speed levels due to the elasticity of skin [27], necessitating larger insertion forces. The stem portion of the microneedles affects the total insertion forces due to the frictional interactions between the microneedles and skin tissue. *Bevel angle* affects both the insertion and retention (i.e., keeping MNAs in place after inserting into the skin tissue) [26]. *Fillet radius* at the base of the microneedles help reduce the stress concentration, thereby increasing the strength of microneedles [24, 26]. *Tip-to-tip distance* controls the MNA skin-piercing event. When the microneedles are placed too close to one another, either the piercing does not occur or high piercing forces are required [23–25]. This is due to what is referred to as the *bed of nails effect*. Furthermore, higher needle density may considerably reduce the total penetration volume (and thus the delivery amount) [23, 25]. In addition to the aforementioned individual effects of each geometric parameter, the array geometry controls the stress distribution on the MNA, the maximum deliverable biocargo amount, and the initial tissue damage resulting from the insertion of the MNAs into the skin.

Apart from the aforementioned geometric aspects of MNAs, innovative microneedle and array designs may be realized by introducing various advanced features (Figure 3.3), including: (1) *conformable MNAs:* MNAs with a flexible backing layer (Figure 3.3a) that can enable conformal contact between the MNA and the complex topography of the underlying skin to enhance the penetration and delivery performance [28]; and (2) *layer-loaded MNAs* (as opposed to uniformly distributed bioactive cargo; see Figure 3.3b): MNAs with controlled location of the biocargo within the microneedles and across the array that can enable improved spatial control and delivery efficiency to targeted skin microenvironments (Figures 3.3c and 3.3d show multilayer-loaded and tip-loaded MNAs, respectively). This selective layer loading has yet to be exploited in the literature other than localizing the drug at the tip of microneedles [30–32]. Furthermore, multiple bioactive cargoes can be loaded into or onto the MNAs, and then delivered simultaneously to targeted skin microenvironments for novel skin-targeted immunization and treatment strategies [33].

Myriad microneedle geometries, comprising cylindrical [34], rectangular [35], pyramidal [26], conical [19], obelisk [24, 26], and negative bevel obelisk [24, 26], with different microneedle lengths and widths, have been developed (Figure 3.4) [6]. Typical geometries vary from 100 μm to 1500 μm in length, from 50 μm to 1000 μm in base width, and from 1 μm to 40 μm in tip diameter [6, 36].

The insertion of a microneedle into a tissue involves six distinct phases: (1) pre-penetration; (2) initial piercing; (3) progressing head penetration; (4) complete head penetration; (5) stem penetration; and

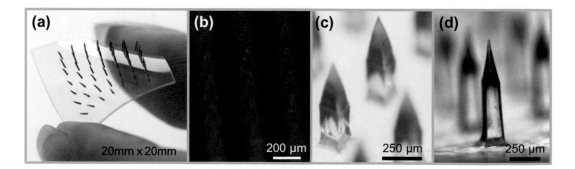

FIGURE 3.3 Innovative microneedle and array designs toward application-oriented optimization. **(a)** Conformable MNAs with a flexible backing layer (reproduced with permission [28]). Selective layer-loaded MNAs: **(b)** Uniformly loaded microneedles (reproduced with permission [29]), **(c)** layer-loaded microneedles (unpublished work from the Ozdoganlar lab at Carnegie Mellon University), and **(d)** tip-loaded microneedles (reproduced with permission [30]).

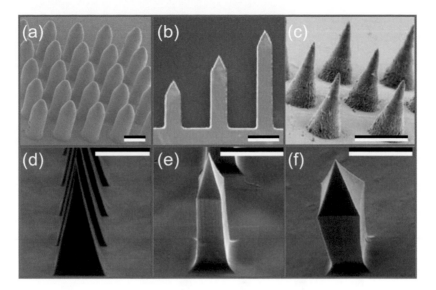

FIGURE 3.4 Different microneedle stem geometries. **(a)** Cylindrical (reproduced with permission [34]), **(b)** Rectangular (reproduced with permission [35]), **(c)** Conical (reproduced with permission [19]), **(d)** Pyramidal (reproduced with permission [26]), **(e)** Obelisk (reproduced with permission [26]), **(f)** Negative obelisk (reproduced with permission [26]). Scale bars correspond to 300 μm.

(6) final tissue relaxation. Depending on the microneedle and array geometries, insertion conditions (e.g., insertion speed), and tissue characteristics, some of these phases may not exist or may not be distinguishable. For instance, for a pyramidal needle, phases 4 and 5 are not present since the overall geometry is smooth without a head-stem transition. On the other hand, phase 2 may not be recognizable when a very sharp (small tip radius) needle penetrates into a very elastic tissue. This dependence on the needle geometry and tissue properties has led different works in the literature (e.g., ref. [37]) to identify different selections of insertion phases. Since an obelisk microneedle shape (see Figure 3.2b) embodies many of geometric features and could show all different phases, we will consider this shape in describing the forces.

The forces associated with the six insertion phases are schematically presented in Figure 3.5. The *pre-penetration phase* begins when the microneedle tip comes into contact with the skin tissue. As the microneedle is pushed further, the skin tissue deforms elastically, and an associated increase in forces is observed. The duration of pre-penetration phase depends on the tip sharpness and tissue properties, the latter of which might change considerably depending on the penetration speed (viscoelasticity and dynamic response) and the tissue preparation (e.g., stretching). Commonly, the sharper the microneedle tip and the lower the effective tissue elasticity, the shorter the pre-penetration phase. This phase will conclude with the *initial piercing phase*, when the tissue surface is punctured. In this short phase, the microneedle tip will penetrate the tissue, and some of the elastic (strain) energy will be released, causing a drop in the insertion forces.

During the *progressing head penetration phase*, the forces will steadily increase. These forces include continued "cutting" force at the microneedle tip and forces caused by the steady expansion of the punctured tissue area due to increasing cross-sectional area of the microneedle head. This increase in forces continues until the punctured tissue area reaches the area of the stem, that is, when the *complete head penetration phase* is reached. In this short phase, another relaxation event will occur, and a sharp drop in the insertion forces will be recognized.

As the microneedle is further inserted into the tissue, the stem penetration phase marked with a steady increase in forces is observed. These forces arise from the shear stresses (causing frictional forces on the microneedle) between the tissue and the microneedle stem. The force will continue to increase with the increased needle depth, until the penetration is stopped. At this point, *the final tissue relaxation phase*, which is characterized by the force relaxation due to strain energy release, will occur [38, 39].

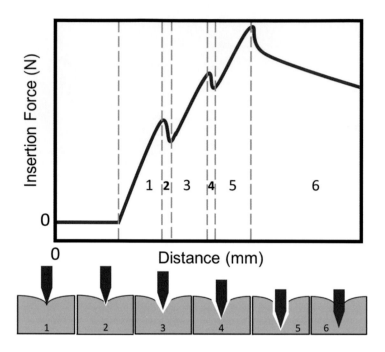

FIGURE 3.5   A typical needle-tissue insertion force diagram [71].

In summary, microneedle and array designs play a crucial role in the tissue penetration and insertion forces. For instance, blunt and short needles, or needles that are too closely spaced in the array, may cause the skin to fold around the needles, limiting or hindering the penetration capability. Weaker microneedle materials, non-optimal MNA designs, and unfavorable insertion conditions might result in excessive insertion forces, and the associated stress levels might exceed the strength of the microneedle material, resulting in mechanical failure of the microneedles. This being so, microneedle and array geometries are critical factors in developing clinically relevant MNA-based drug delivery systems. Comprehensive models that capture the effects of microneedle and array designs, as well as accurate skin tissue characteristics, could facilitate optimization of MNA-based drug delivery strategies. Developing such models requires a thorough understanding of the relationships between microneedle/array designs and insertion forces, and of the key mechanical properties of the skin.

3.3 Microneedle-Manufacturing Techniques

This section summarizes the current fabrication approaches of both the coated and dissolvable MNAs, as well as the coating methods toward satisfying key requirements in developing clinically relevant MNAs.

Successful manufacturing of MNAs is of utmost importance for their regulatory approval and clinical adaption. An effective manufacturing technique for both the coated and the dissolvable MNAs should satisfy certain key requirements, including (1) *accuracy and reproducibility*, yielding dimensionally accurate MNAs encapsulating a precise dosage of biocargo; (2) *material applicability*, which entails capability to use a broad range of relevant materials for MNAs so that optimal insertion and delivery performance for different vaccines and therapeutics is obtained without any toxic effects and unwanted immune response; (3) *geometric capability*, which enables creating required microneedle and array geometries toward optimal insertion and delivery performance; (4) *benign processing*, that is, processing without toxic chemical solvents or high temperatures that can damage the bioactive cargo; and (5) *low cost and scalability*, which is required for the process to be used for commercial applications in terms of production cost and volume. Furthermore, an ideal fabrication approach should facilitate easy, rapid, and low-cost changes in geometric and material parameters for optimization.

The existing microneedle manufacturing approaches can be classified into two main categories: (a) direct fabrication techniques and (b) hybrid fabrication techniques, which involve a direct fabrication technique followed by the use of a micromolding method [26, 36, 70].

3.3.1 Direct Fabrication Techniques

Direct fabrication techniques used for solid MNAs include photolithography [21], laser cutting [35], micromachining [26], and additive manufacturing (i.e., 3D printing) [40]. Photolithographic processes are among the first microneedle manufacturing methods for reproducible fabrication of accurate solid MNAs. However, the use of photolithography-based approaches for MNA fabrication imposes strict material (e.g., silicon, silicon-oxides, and a few metals) and geometric limitations, requires a long time from conception to fabrication, and occasions high production costs for small-to-medium production volumes. Specialized cleanroom processing, use of hazardous chemicals, and expensive production equipment are other disadvantages. These requirements and shortcomings hinder rapid and low-cost fabrication of different MNA designs, limiting the capability to conduct parametric studies for optimization of microneedle and array designs [26, 31].

Laser-based approaches (e.g., laser UV cutting) are also used to fabricate the solid MNAs from thermoplastic polymers and metals [35]. Even though these methods can effectively create MNAs, they usually suffer from poor geometric integrity, low dimensional accuracy, low surface quality, and large form errors (e.g., blunt tips) due to the process generated heat and residual stresses. Laser-based approaches also impose further geometric restrictions since they are limited to fabricating planar (i.e., 2.5D) features rather than fully 3D features.

Mechanical micromachining (e.g., micromilling) has recently emerged as an effective manufacturing technique for MNAs [26]. An important advantage of this technology is its capacity to generate any microscale geometry on a range of materials, including polymers, metals, and ceramics, in a highly reproducible and accurate fashion [26]. The lead time for fabricating new designs is measured in minutes or hours, and the unit cost of the parts created by micromilling is very low. Most recently, a diamond micromilling approach has been introduced to further advance micromachining-based solid MNA (including master mold) fabrication [26, 31]. Therefore, the use of micromilling could address the aforementioned shortcomings of photolithography- and laser-based microneedle fabrication processes (especially during the design optimization stages) in geometric and material capability, cost, and ramp-up time [26].

More recently, additive manufacturing and 3D printing approaches have been adapted for fabricating MNA-based trans/intradermal drug delivery systems. For example, a two-photon-initiated polymerization method was demonstrated for fabricating MNAs, where a near-infrared ultrashort-pulsed laser was focused into a photocurable resin to create the 3D microneedles using a layer-by-layer approach [41]. However, currently, 3D printing brings limitations in material capability, achievable resolution, and scalability. Further advancements in 3D printing might enable more innovative microneedle and array designs toward application-oriented optimizations.

The direct fabrication techniques are not restricted by the geometrical constraints arising from the micromolding step of the hybrid fabrication techniques, and thus are capable of creating more innovative microneedle designs, such as those with undercuts [42–44]. On the other hand, the direct fabrication techniques suffer from one or more drawbacks that prevent high-throughput industrial manufacturing of MNAs, including limited production rates and high costs for scaling up to higher production volumes.

3.3.2 Hybrid Fabrication Techniques

Hybrid fabrication techniques can be utilized to create both coated and dissolvable MNAs. The general approach in hybrid fabrication techniques involves fabrication of a set of master molds using a direct technique, and subsequently using micromolding to create the final MNAs. The MNAs can be fabricated using micromolding either directly from the master molds or from production molds obtained from the master molds. Silicon, metals (e.g., aluminum), and thermoplastic polymers (e.g., poly(methyl methacrylate), PMMA) have been used as master mold materials [26, 45]. The molds (master or production) are filled with a molten, dissolved (solvent-based), multi-component (e.g., thermosets) or softened (above the glass-transition temperature) material to create solid polymer microneedles upon solidification (by cooling, solvent evaporation, or cross-linking). Similarly, ceramic microneedles have been fabricated by molding a ceramic-powder slurry (e.g., alumina) onto the MNA molds, and then sintering the molded slurry [47].

3.3.3 Fabrication of Coated MNAs

Coated MNAs are obtained by coating the solid MNAs, created using either the direct or the hybrid fabrication techniques, with the desired biocargo (Figure 3.6a) [45–47]. The coating process commonly involves dipping the non-dissolvable (solid) MNAs into a liquid solution of a bioactive molecules, or spraying the solution onto the solid MNAs [6, 36]. Alternatively, a layer-by-layer coating approach has also been demonstrated in the literature [48].

The solution with bioactive molecules is often prepared so that its viscosity is sufficient to conformally spread onto the microneedles during drying [6, 36, 46]. A biocompatible surfactant is usually added to the coating formulation to facilitate the wetting of the microneedle surface [6, 49]. A stabilizing polymer may be used to protect the biocargo from damage during drying and storage [6, 49]. The amount of biocargo that will be coated is adjusted by controlling the initial concentration of the drug solution. For relatively higher doses, since the coating solution may become too viscous, desired drug dose is obtained by applying multiple coating steps. The coating solution is formulated for optimal delivery performance, such as dissolution of coating within the desired time period after penetrating the skin. In addition to applying them to the entire microneedle, when the required doses are sufficiently low coatings might be localized just to the microneedle tips, to increase the delivery efficiency. Alternatively, if the coating makes the tips very blunt, diminishing the insertion performance of MNAs, only the shafts might be

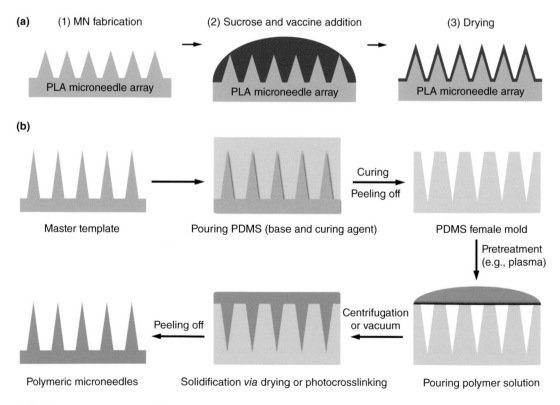

FIGURE 3.6 Manufacturing of **(a)** coated (reproduced with permission [45]) and **(b)** dissolvable MNAs (reproduced with permission [46]).

coated. Using benign conditions during the coating and drying steps is critical to maintaining the activity of the biocargo, especially for the heat-sensitive drugs.

3.3.4 Fabrication of Dissolvable MNAs

Dissolvable MNAs are fabricated from biodissolvable materials. The biocargo is incorporated into the biodissolvable material, dissolution of which within the skin facilitates precise delivery of the biocargo. Commonly, dissolvable MNAs are created using a hybrid fabrication technique: As depicted in Figure 3.6b, the general approach involves manufacturing the master molds using a direct fabrication approach, fabricating the production or female molds with the microneedle-shaped wells using elastomer molding, and creating the final dissolvable MNAs using a micromolding technique (e.g., injection molding [50], investment molding [51], spin-casting [21, 26, 67–71], and pouring [52]). In a few studies (e.g., ref. [19]), laser-based techniques were used to directly fabricate the elastomer production molds with the microneedle-shaped wells.

The bioactive cargo incorporated into the hydrogel microneedle matrix is commonly distributed uniformly within the entire microneedle (Figure 3.3b). More recently, concentrating the bioactive cargo only at the tips, or more generally, loading one or more bioactive cargoes in different locations of the microneedle has been demonstrated (e.g., layer-loaded MNAs in Figure 3.3c) [30, 31]. The *tip or layer-loaded MNAs* have potential to bring further advances for effective skin immunization and therapy strategies. However, there are still important challenges in accurate, reproducible, and controllable fabrication of these MNAs, and thus a strong need to further develop effective manufacturing approaches.

The most commonly used micromolding technique for creating dissolvable MNAs has been spin-casting, since it not only satisfies many of the aforementioned key manufacturing requirements, but also is relatively simple, low-cost, and scalable. The spin-casting technique has been applied to a broad range of biodissolvable materials with myriad biocargoes [21, 26]. Importantly, its low-temperature processing capability enables maintaining the activity of heat-sensitive biologics. The first step in the technique is to fabricate high-accuracy microneedle molds. This can be done either by directly creating the production molds [19] or by creating a master mold [21, 26] that can then be replicated to obtain many production molds. Each production mold can then be used to create a large number of dissolvable MNAs through the spin-casting approach. Due to the nature of solvent-based casting, a certain amount of shrinkage is observed in the dissolvable MNAs due to the drying process. However, for a given geometry, the amount of shrinkage is consistent, resulting in reproducible geometries [26]. Yet prediction of the shrinkage behavior for different process conditions is critical to fabricating accurate and reproducible MNAs.

For the MNA materials they can produce, the hybrid fabrication techniques can address many of the drawbacks of the direct fabrication techniques for creating the final MNAs. The hybrid fabrication techniques hold the potential to be a predictable, reproducible, inexpensive, accurate, and scalable approach for fabricating MNAs. To realize these attractive benefits, further advances are needed to precisely control geometric and mechanical properties of the MNAs, and to enable fabrication of clinically relevant MNA designs.

3.4 Microneedle Materials

The microneedle materials are critical for both effective penetration and cargo delivery performance of MNAs. Furthermore, the effects of microneedle materials on the bioactivity and longevity/stability of the MNA-embedded biocargo should be carefully considered.

For both the coated and the dissolvable microneedles, the choice of material directly affects the mechanical strength and biocompatibility [23, 53, 26, 71]. Furthermore, the choice of dissolvable material and coating formulation strongly impact the drug delivery profile, including intradermal release kinetics and intradermal residence of the delivered drugs. Importantly, the microneedle material should preserve the viability of the incorporated biocargoes, and should enable satisfying the desired storage duration without affecting the bioactivity of the biocargoes. Therefore, favorable biocompatible materials should be identified or formulated toward optimized clinical applications and long-term stability of the MNA-integrated biocargoes.

3.4.1 Materials for Coated MNAs

As mentioned above, coated MNAs utilize solid, non-dissolvable microneedles coated by a layer of aqueous solution incorporating the relevant bioactive cargo. Coated microneedles have been fabricated from a number of materials, including silicon [54]; many metals, such as stainless steel [35] and titanium [55]; non-dissolvable polymers (e.g., a copolymer of methylvinyl/ether and maleic anhydride (PMVE/MA) [56], poly-L-lactic acid (PLA) [45], and polymethylmethacrylate (PMMA) [57]); and ceramics [58]. Despite promising results obtained using those materials, materials with better inertness and biocompatibility are still needed to implement clinically relevant MNA designs. To elaborate, since the coated MNAs utilize non-dissolvable microneedles, it is imperative that the needles remain fully intact during the insertion and removal to prevent any complications that can arise from material residue left in the skin. Biocompatibility of the structural material and coating formulation is also critical to avert any adverse immunologic or toxic effects arising from the dissolution of the coating layer.

In general, the coating formulations should account for the following considerations: (1) Controlled spreading of the coating solution onto the microneedles to obtain uniform coating of the microneedle surfaces. Specifically, the increased viscosity and reduced contact angle between the aqueous coating solution and the microneedle surfaces can improve the wetting and, in turn, the coating performance. (2) The coating formulation should be water-soluble to enable the coating process and to ensure rapid and complete dissolution of the coating in the skin microenvironment. (3) The mechanical strength of the dried coating on the needle surfaces should be sufficient to keep the coating adhered to them during insertion. (4) The coating solution should be biologically safe, and formulated such that the activity of the biocargo is maintained during both drying and storage [6, 49]. The water-soluble solution of the biocargo is often formulated at a sufficiently high viscosity to enable better retention on the microneedle surfaces during drying [6, 49]. To further improve the coating performance, surfactants that facilitate enhanced wetting of the surface may be used [49]. Stabilizing polymers may be added to the coating formulation to protect the biocargo during both drying and storage [6].

To formulate an effective coating with a broad range of bioactive cargoes, a myriad of water-soluble biomaterials have been used [6, 49]. The most commonly used biodissolvable polymers include carboxymethylcellulose (CMC) [35], sucrose [49], sodium alginate [49], hyaluronic acid (HA) [49], glycerol [49], poly(lactic-co-glycolic acid) (PLGA) [49], and polyvinylpyrrolidone (PVP) [49]. To further improve the coating performance, surfactants, such as Poloxamer 188 [41], Lutrol F-68 NF [35], and Quil-A [41] have been used. In addition, stabilizers, such as trehalose, sucrose, glucose, and dextrans have been used to maintain the biological activity of the drugs during the coating process and subsequent storage [6, 48, 59]. The same stabilizing agents can be added to the materials of dissolvable materials [60].

3.4.2 Materials for Dissolvable MNAs

Dissolvable MNAs are specifically designed to completely dissolve in the skin, thereby leaving no biohazardous waste or sharps after use. Most dissolving microneedles in the literature need to remain in skin for at least 5 min to fully dissolve. If controlled-release performance is desired, biodegradable polymer microneedles might be designed to achieve a defined dissolution profile and remain in the skin for extended periods (e.g., days). As a general rule, dissolvable MNAs should be fabricated from biologically safe [69], water-soluble materials that will dissolve in the skin after insertion. While dissolving microneedles might be used as a skin pretreatment to increase permeability, drugs are often encapsulated inside the needle for release into the skin similarly to coated microneedles.

Biodissolvable and biodegradable MNAs that incorporate the bioactive cargo have been fabricated using hybrid techniques for a range of biocompatible polymers (singly or in combination), including poly-L-lactic acid (PLA) [61, 62], poly-glycolic acid (PGA) [61], poly-lactic-co-glycolic acid (PLGA) [14, 61], poly(vinylpyrrolidone) (PVP) [20, 26], poly(vinyl) alcohol (PVA) [19], CMC [21, 26, 31], and silk [63], as well as sugars, including galactose [64], dextrin [64], and maltose [26].

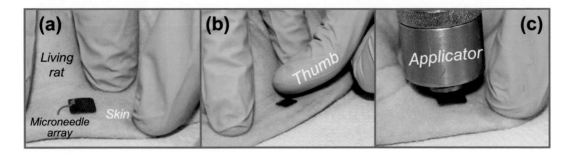

FIGURE 3.7 Microneedle administration to living rats: **(a)** A microneedle array placed on living rat skin; **(b)** Thumb insertion; and **(c)** Device-assisted application [The Ozdoganlar group at Carnegie Mellon University, unpublished].

3.5 MNA Administration Methods

A critical step toward enabling clinical adaptation of MNA-based trans/intradermal delivery systems is to ensure that each administration of MNAs precisely delivers the required dose in a minimally invasive manner. Therefore, MNAs should be capable of piercing the SC layer of skin with minimal force and obtaining the desired penetration depths in a reproducible manner. However, inherent elasticity and complex topography of skin, combined with the micron-scale-size microneedles, pose challenges for precise and reproducible delivery using MNAs (Figure 3.7a).

Unlike the conventional transdermal patches, MNAs require an external force to facilitate effective and reproducible penetration of microneedles into the skin [21, 65]. This external force can be provided either by a manual application method (i.e., thumb insertion, Figure 3.7b) or by using an external application device (i.e., an applicator, Figure 3.7c). Although it has been demonstrated that long microneedles with sharp tips can be manually inserted into skin, obtaining uniform insertion forces, achieving consistent penetration depths is very challenging [50, 65]. On the other hand, an applicator can control the insertion speed (and thus, the insertion force), thereby enabling reproducible penetration into the skin [53, 65]. For this reason, applicators are preferred over manual application. The devices can be for either single or multiple use.

A few studies have highlighted the necessity of an applicator. Crichton et al. [66] showed that, by varying the application speed of coated microneedles, the piercing depth and the delivered dose can be increased. Applicators are especially needed for high-density, short MNAs with blunt microneedles to ensure a sufficient penetration depth [23, 27]. Verbaan et al. [27] showed that although manual application failed to enable 300-μm-long microneedles to pierce the skin, such needles successfully and reproducibly pierced the skin when an external applicator was used. Increasing the applicator speed commonly improves penetration (i.e., enables a larger needle portion to penetrate). However, beyond a certain speed, applicators may increase the chance of damage to the dermal and/or subdermal tissues. Therefore, an optimal penetration speed should be identified for a given microneedle and array geometry and skin properties.

When designing applicator devices for clinical use, a number of design criteria should be met. Since a major benefit of MNAs is to improve patient compliance by eliminating pain, the use of the applicator should be pain-free. Furthermore, the applicator should enable more reproducible and controlled administration of MNAs without increasing the risk of mechanical failure of MNAs. Considering the wide range of microneedle designs and skin conditions, advancing the applicator designs and identifying optimal penetration conditions through microneedle insertion studies are critical for the clinical adaptation of MNAs.

3.6 Conclusions and Outlook

Microneedle-based drug delivery systems, which are enabled by recent advances in microfabrication technologies, could bring exciting advances to transdermal drug delivery. Microneedle arrays with coated or dissolvable needles are among the most popular microneedle concepts developed in recent years, and pharmaceutical companies have shown a great interest in these technologies. However, the true potential of coated or dissolvable MNA-based drug delivery has yet to be achieved due to considerable challenges in design, manufacturing, and administration of MNAs. Many design, manufacturing, and administration requirements must be addressed to create clinically applicable MNA-based transdermal drug delivery systems.

This chapter presented an overview on the design, fabrication, and administration of the coated and dissolvable MNAs. The design (i.e., both the geometry and the material) of the needles controls their skin penetration and biocargo delivery performance. The material also affects the bioactivity and longevity of the biocargo incorporated into or onto the needles. Further studies are needed to identify optimal geometries and materials for achieving clinically applicable and reproducible delivery of a broad range of therapeutics and vaccines using MNAs.

The fabrication technique used for creating the MNAs dictates both the attainable geometries and the utilizable materials for the MNAs. To be effective, a manufacturing technique should be capable of reproducibly creating MNAs with diverse geometries and from a myriad of biomaterials. In addition, the scalability of the fabrication technique directly affects the cost of the microneedle-based drug delivery systems. Moreover, manufacturing conditions could have a strong influence on the stability and viability of the drugs when they are coated onto or integrated within the MNAs. Therefore, development of scalable, controllable, and cost-effective approaches for MNA manufacturing is fundamental to realizing further advances in MNA-based delivery systems toward their clinical deployment.

Successful MNA administration entails piercing of the SC and achieving the desired penetration depths in a reproducible manner. To this end, the application method, including manual or device-assisted approaches, plays a critical role. Further research is needed for identifying application methods and associated conditions for satisfactory administration of MNAs. When addressing these objectives, the skin properties, which may vary throughout the body and change from person to person, should also be considered.

Taken together, MNAs show great promise of significantly advancing the existing administration techniques for transdermal and intradermal delivery of biocargoes, and of bringing exciting new therapies and immunization strategies. However, further research into MNA design, manufacturing, materials, and administration is needed for realizing clinically applicable MNA-based drug delivery systems. Effectively addressing those aspects are also prerequisites to regulatory approval of MNAs by various government agencies.

REFERENCES

1. Prausnitz MR, Langer R. Transdermal drug delivery. Nature Biotechnology. 2012; 26(11):1261–1268.
2. Donnelly RF, Singh TRR, Woolfson AD. Microneedle-based drug delivery systems: Microfabrication, drug delivery, and safety. Drug Delivery. 2010; 17(4):187–207.
3. Hedge NR, Kaveri SV, Bayry J. Recent advances in the administration of vaccines for infectious diseases: Microneedles as painless delivery devices for mass vaccination. Drug Discovery Today. 2011; 16(1–2):1061–1068.
4. Arora A, Prausnitz MR, Mitragotri S. Micro-scale devices for transdermal drug delivery. International Journal of Pharmaceutics. 2008; 364(2):227–236.
5. Bouwstra JA. The skin barrier, a well-organized membrane. Colloids and Surfaces A: Physicochemical and Engineering Aspects. 1997; 123:403–413.
6. Kim YC, Park JH, Prausnitz MR. Microneedles for drug and vaccine delivery. Advanced Drug Delivery Reviews. 2012; 64(14):1547–1568.
7. Walker RB, Smith EW. The role of percutaneous penetration enhancers. Advanced Drug Delivery Reviews. 1996; 18(3):295–301.
8. Nair LS, Laurencin CT. Biodegradable polymers as biomaterials. Progress in Polymer Science. 2007; 32(8–9):762–798.
9. Karande P, Mitragotri S. Enhancement of transdermal drug delivery via synergistic action of chemicals. Biochimica et Biophysica Acta. 2009; 1788(11):2362–2373.
10. Williams AC, Barry BW. Penetration enhancers. Advanced Drug Delivery Reviews. 2004; 56(5):128–137.
11. Shivanand P, Binal P, Viral D, Shaliesh K, Manish G, Subhash V. Microneedle: Various techniques of fabrications and evaluations. International Journal of ChemTech Research. 2009; 1(4):1058–1062.

12. Wissink JM, Berenschot JW, Tas NR. Atom sharp microneedles, the missing link in microneedle drug delivery. In Proceedings of Medical Devices Conference. 2008.

13. Gill H, Denson D, Burris B. Effect of microneedle design on pain in human subjects. Clinical Journal of Pain. 2008; 24(7):585–594.

14. Jain RA. The manufacturing techniques of various drug loaded biodegradable poly(lactide-co-glycolide) (PLGA) devices. Biomaterials. 2000; 21(23):2475–2090.

15. Ma G. Wu C. Microneedle, bio-microneedle and bio-inspired microneedle: A review. Journal of Controlled Release. 2017; 251:11–23.

16. Nordquist L, Roxhed N, Griss P, Stemme G. Novel microneedle patches for active insulin delivery are efficient in maintaining glycaemic control: An initial comparison with subcutaneous administration. Pharmaceutical Research. 2007; 24(7):1381–1388.

17. Roxhed N, Gasser T, Griss P. Penetration-enhanced ultra-sharp microneedles and prediction on skin interaction for efficient transdermal drug delivery. Journal of Microelectromechanical Systems. 2007; 16(6):1429–1440.

18. Koutsonanos DG, Pilar MMD, Zarnitsyn VG, Sullivan SP, Compans RW, Prausnitz MR. Transdermal influenza immunization with vaccine-coated microneedle arrays. PloS One. 2009; 4(3): e4773.

19. Donnelly RF, Majithiya R, Singh TRR, Morrow DIJ, Garland MJ, Demir YK, et al. Design, optimization and characterisation of polymeric microneedle arrays prepared by a novel laser-based micromoulding technique. Pharmaceutical Research. 2011; 28(1):41–57.

20. Sullivan SP, Murthy N, Prausnitz MR. Minimally invasive protein delivery with rapidly dissolving polymer microneedles. Advanced Materials. 2008; 20(5):933–938.

21. Lee JW, Park J, Prausnitz MR. Dissolving microneedles for transdermal drug delivery. Biomaterials. 2008; 29(13):2113–2124.

22. Gardeniers HJGE, Luttge R, Berenschot EJW, De Boer MJ, Yeshurun SY, Hefetz MS, et al. Silicon micromachined hollow microneedles for transdermal liquid transport. Journal of Microelectromechanical Systems. 2003; 12(6):855–862.

23. Prausnitz MR. Engineering microneedle patches for vaccination and drug delivery to skin. Annual Review of Chemical and Biomolecular Engineering. 2017; 8:9.1–9.2.

24. Falo LD, Erdos G, Ozdoganlar OB. Dissolvable microneedle arrays for transdermal delivery to human skin. Patent No. US 2011/0098651 A1, USA. 2011.

25. Donnelly RF, Garland MJ, Morrow DIJ, Migalska K, Singh TRR, Majithiya R, et al. Optical coherence tomography is a valuable tool in the study of the effects of microneedle geometry on skin penetration characteristics and in-skin dissolution. Journal of Controlled Release. 2010; 147(3):333–341.

26. Bediz, Bekir, Emrullah Korkmaz, Rakesh Khilwani, Cara Donahue, Geza Erdos, Louis D. Falo, and O. Burak Ozdoganlar. "Dissolvable microneedle arrays for intradermal delivery of biologics: fabrication and application." *Pharmaceutical research* 31, no. 1 (2014): 117–135.

27. Verbaan FJ, Bal SM, Berg DJV, Dijksman JAD, Hecke MV, Verpoorten H, et al. Improved piercing of microneedle arrays in dermatomed human skin by an impact insertion method. Journal of Controlled Release. 2008; 128(1):80–88.

28. Rajabi M, Roxhed N, Shafagh RZ, Haraldson T, Fischer AC, Wijngaart WVD, et al. Flexible and stretchable microneedle patches with integrated rigid stainless steel microneedles for transdermal biointerfacing. Plos One. 2016; 0166330.

29. Moga KA, Bickford LR, Geil RD, Dunn SS, Pandya AA, Wang Y, et al. Rapidly-dissolvable microneedle patches via a highly-scalable and reproducible soft lithography approach. Advanced Materials. 2013; 25(36):5060–5066.

30. Falo LD, Erdos G, Ozdoganlar OB. Tip-loaded microneedle arrays for transdermal insertion. Patent No. US 2015/0126923 A1, USA. 2015.

31. Korkmaz E, Friedrich EE, Ramadan M, Erdos G, Mathers AR, Ozdoganlar OB, et al. Therapeutic intradermal delivery of tumor necrosis factor-alpha antibodies using tip-loaded dissolvable microneedle arrays. Acta Biomaterialia. 2015; 24:96–105.

32. Kim JY, Han MR, Kim YH, Shin SW, Nam SY, Park JH. Tip-loaded dissolving microneedles for transdermal delivery of donepezil hydrochloride for treatment of Alzheimer's disease. European Journal of Pharmaceutics and Biopharmaceutics. 2016; 105:148–155.

33. Lau S, Fei J, Liu H, Chen W, Liu R. Multilayered pyramidal dissolving microneedle patches with flexible pedestals for improving effective drug delivery. Journal of Controlled Release. 2017; 265:113–119.

34. Lu Y, Mantha SN, Crowder DC, Chinchilla S, Shah KN, Yun YH, et al. Microstereolithography and characterization of poly(propylene fumarate)-based drug-loaded microneedle arrays. Biofabrication. 2015; 7:045001.

35. Gill HS, Prausnitz MR. Coated microneedles for transdermal delivery. Journal of Controlled Release. 2007; 117(2):227–237.

36. Indermun S, Luttge R, Choonara YE, Kumar P, Toit LCD, Modi G, et al. Current advances in the fabrication of microneedles for transdermal delivery. Journal of Controlled Release. 2014; 185:130–138.

37. Gerwen DJV, Dankelman J, Dobbelsteen JJVD. Needle-tissue interaction forces—A survey of experimental data. Medical Engineering&Physics. 2012; 34:665–680.

38. Barnett AC, Lee YS, Moore JZ. Fracture mechanics model of needle cutting tissue. Journal of Manufacturing Science Engineering. 2015; 138(1):011005.

39. Yang Chongiun, Xie Y, Liu S, Sun D. Force modeling, identification, and feedback control of robot-assisted needle insertion: A survey of the literature. Sensors. 2018; 18(2):561.

40. Pere CPP, Economidou SN, Lall G, Ziraud C, Boateng JS, Alexander BD, et al. 3D printed microneedles for insulin skin delivery. International Journal of Pharmaceutics. 2018; 544(2):425–432.

41. Ovsianikov A, Chichkov B, Mente P, Monterio-Riviere NA, Doraiswamy A, Narayan RJ, et al. Two photon polymerization of polymer-ceramic hybrid materials for transdermal drug delivery. International Journal of Applied Ceramic Technology. 2007; 4:22–29.

42. Filiz S, Xie L, Weiss L, Ozdoganlar OB. Micromilling of microbarbs for medical implants. International Journal of Machine Tools and Manufacture. 2008; 48(3–4):459–472.

43. Xie L, Brownridge SD, Ozdoganlar OB, Weiss LE. The viability of micromilling for manufacturing mechanical attachment components for medical applications. Transactions of NAMRI/SME. 2006; 445–452.

44. Johnson AR, Caudill CL, Tumbleston JR, Bloomquist CJ, Moga KA, Ermoshkin A, et al. Single-step fabrication of computationally designed microneedles by continuous liquid interface production. PloS one. 2016; 11(9); e0162518.

45. DeMuth PC, Li AV, Abbink P, Liu J, Li H, Stanley KA, et al. Vaccine delivery with microneedle skin patches in nonhuman primates. Nature Biotechnology. 2013; 31(12):1082–1085.

46. Wang M, Hu L, Xu C. Recent advances in the design of polymeric microneedles for transdermal drug delivery and biosensing. Lab Chip. 2017; 17:1373–1387.

47. Boks MA, Unger WWJ, Engels S, Abrosini M, Kyook YV, Luttge R. Controlled release of a model vaccine by nanoporous ceramic microneedle arrays. International Journal of Pharmaceutics. 2015; 491(1–2):375–383.

48. Saurer EM, Flessner RM, Sullivan SP, Prausnitz MR, Lynn DM. Layer-by-layer assembly of DNA- and protein-containing films on microneedles for drug delivery to the skin. Biomacromolecules. 2010; 11:3136–3143.

49. Gill HS, Prausnitz MR. Coating formulations for microneedles. Pharmaceutical Research. 2007; 24(7):1369–1380.

50. Sammoura F, Kang J, Heo YM, Jung T, Lin L. Polymeric microneedle fabrication using a microinjection molding technique. Microsystem Technologies. 2006; 13:517–22.

51. Lippmann JM, Geiger EJ, Pisano AP. Polymer investment molding: Method for fabricating hollow, microscale parts. Sensors Actuators A: Physical. 2007; 134:2–10.

52. Yin Z, Kuang D, Wang S, Zheng Z, Yadavalli VK, Lu S. Swellable silk fibroin microneedles for transdermal drug delivery. International Journal of Biological Macromolecules. 2018; 106:48–56.

53. Maaden KVD, Jiskoot W, Bouwstra J. Microneedle technologies for (trans)dermal drug and vaccine delivery. Journal of Controlled Release. 2012; 161:645–655.

54. McGrath MG, Vrdoljak A, O'Mahony C, Oliveira JC, Moore AC, Crean AM. Determination of parameters for successful spray coating of silicon microneedle arrays. International Journal of Pharmaceutics. 2011; 415:140–149.

55. Larraneta E, Lutton REM, Woolfson AD, Donnelly RF. Microneedle arrays as transdermal and intradermal drug delivery systems: Materials science, manufacture and commercial development. Materials Science and Engineering: R: Reports. 2016; 104:1–32.

56. Carmel M, Salvador EC, Fallows SJ, McCarthy HO, Donnelly RF. Microneedle-mediated delivery donepezil: Potential for improved treatment options in Alzheimer's disease. European Journal of Pharmaceutics and Biopharmaceutics. 2016; 103:43–50.

57. Choi SO, Kim YC, Park JH, Hutcheson J, Gill HS, Yoon YK, et al. An electrically active microneedle array for electroporation. Biomedical Microdevices. 2010; 12(2):263–273.

58. Cai B, Xia W, Bredenberg S, Li H, Enggyist H. Bioceramic microneedles with flexible and self-swelling substrate. European Journal of Pharmaceutics and Biopharmaceutics. 2015; 94:404–410.

59. Kim YC, ShiQuan F, Compans RW, MooKang S, Prausnitz MR. Formulation and coating of microneedles with inactivated influenza virus to improve vaccine stability and immunogenicity. Journal of Controlled Release. 2010; 142 (2):187–195.

60. Bachy V, Hervouet C, Becker PD, Chorro L, Carlin LM, Herath S, et al. Langerin negative dendritic cells promote potent CD8+ T-cell priming by skin delivery of live adenovirus vaccine microneedle arrays. PNAS. 2013; 110(8):3041–3046.

61. Park JH, Allen MG, Prausnitz MR. Biodegradable polymer microneedles: Fabrication, mechanics and transdermal drug delivery. Journal of Control Release. 2005; 104(1):51–66.

62. Park JH, Allen MG, Prausnitz MR. Polymer microneedles for controlled-release drug delivery. Pharmaceutical Research. 2006; 23(5):1008–1019.

63. Tsioris K, Raja WK, Pritchard EM, Panilaitis B, Kaplan DL, Omenetto FG. Fabrication of silk microneedles for controlled- release drug delivery. Advanced Functional Materials. 2012; 22(2):330–335.

64. Donnelly RF, Morrow DIJ, Singh TRR, Migalska K, Mccarron A, Mahony CO, et al. Processing difficulties and instability of carbohydrate microneedle arrays. Drug Development and Industrial Pharmacy. 2009; 35(10):1242–1254.

65. Singh TRR, Dunne NJ, Cunningham E, Donnelly RF. Review of patents on microneedle applicators. Recent Patents on Drug Delivery&Formulation. 2011; 5:11–23.

66. Crichton ML, Ansaldo A, Chen X, Prow TW, Fernando GJP, Kendall MAF. The effect of strain rate on the precision of penetration of short densely- packed microprojection array patches coated with vaccine. Biomaterials. 2010; 31:4562–4572.

67. Korkmaz, E., Friedrich, E.E., Ramadan, M.H., Erdos, G., Mathers, A.R., Ozdoganlar, O.B., et al., 2015 Therapeutic intradermal delivery of tumor necrosis factor-alpha antibodies using tip-loaded dissolvable microneedle arrays. *Acta biomaterialia, 24*, pp.96-105.

68. Korkmaz, E., Friedrich, E.E., Ramadan, M.H., Erdos, G., Mathers, A.R., Ozdoganlar, et al., 2016. Tip-loaded dissolvable microneedle arrays effectively deliver polymer-conjugated antibody inhibitors of tumor-necrosis-factor-alpha into human skin. *Journal of pharmaceutical sciences, 105*(11), pp.3453-3457.

69. Yalcintas, E.P., Ackerman, D.S., Korkmaz, E., Telmer, C.A., Jarvik, J.W., Campbell, P.G., Bruchez, M.P. and Ozdoganlar, O.B., 2020. Analysis of In Vitro Cytotoxicity of Carbohydrate-Based Materials Used for Dissolvable Microneedle Arrays. *Pharmaceutical Research, 37*(3), p.33.

70. Kovaliov, M., Li, S., Korkmaz, E., Cohen-Karni, D., Tomycz, N., Ozdoganlar, O.B. and Averick, S., 2017. Extended-release of opioids using fentanyl-based polymeric nanoparticles for enhanced pain management. *RSC advances, 7*(76), pp.47904–47912.

71. Khilwani, R., Gilgunn, P.J., Kozai, T.D., Ong, X.C., Korkmaz, E., Gunalan, P.K., Cui, X.T., Fedder, G.K. and Ozdoganlar, O.B., 2016. Ultra-miniature ultra-compliant neural probes with dissolvable delivery needles: design, fabrication and characterization. Biomedical microdevices, 18(6), p.97.

4

Hollow Microneedles

Iman Mansoor[1], Boris Stoeber[1,2]
[1] *Department of Electrical and Computer Engineering*
  The University of British Columbia
[2] *Department of Mechanical Engineering*
  The University of British Columbia

4.1 Introduction

Hollow microneedles are much smaller in size but otherwise similar to the conventional needles that have been used with syringes since the 1850s. There are several key differences compared to other microneedles discussed in this book. The hollow lumen with typical inner diameters smaller than 100 μm represents the main challenge to the manufacturing of hollow microneedles. In principle, injectable drugs do not require reformulation for injection through hollow microneedles, given that hollow microneedles provide a conduit for injecting fluids into the body similar to that of conventional hollow needles, providing a relatively simple regulatory path. In addition to fluid injection into the body, several sensing concepts have been developed based on hollow microneedles; these will be discussed in Chapter 8. Here we will focus on the general characteristics of hollow microneedles.

4.2 Fabrication Technology for Hollow Microneedles

Hollow microneedles are fabricated using microelectromechanical systems (MEMS) technology. Fabrication typically starts from a flat substrate such as a silicon or glass wafer using tools originally developed for the integrated circuit (IC) industry and additional more specialized tools. This suggests that hollow microneedles can benefit from the scalability of the underlying technology; however, the long duration of some process steps performed on investment-intensive equipment can be challenging. Unlike IC devices, whose feature sizes keep shrinking leading to shorter process steps, hollow microneedles require large feature sizes due to their application-specific requirements.

The manufacturing strategies for hollow microneedles depend strongly on the orientation of the needle shaft with respect to the substrate plane. It is therefore common practice to classify microneedles with respect to their shaft orientation: that is, as in-plane when the shaft orientation is parallel to the substrate plane and as out-of-plane in the case of a shaft perpendicular to the substrate plane.

4.2.1 In-Plane Microneedles

The earliest hollow microneedles developed in the early 1990s were in-plane designs based on silicon developed using MEMS technology available at that time. Surface micromachining had recently been developed, in which the successive deposition and patterning of thin films of metals, dielectrics, and semiconductors and the removal of so-called sacrificial layers results in microstructures that reside in near proximity of the substrate surface. A technique introduced in the late 1960s used for "bulk-micromachining" takes advantage of the crystal structure of single-crystal silicon wafers through anisotropic etching using etchants such as potassium hydroxide (KOH). The direction-dependent etch rate results in structures defined by particular crystal planes.

Several approaches used silicon as the supporting substrate and provided the flow channel on top or within the silicon substrate. Lin et al. (1) used a combination of surface micromachining and anisotropic silicon wet etching to form single microneedles with a shaft length between 1 and 6 mm. The enclosed flow channel was 9 µm high and 30–50 µm wide. The needles were 70 µm thick and 80–140 µm wide. Paik et al. (2) used a buried-channel technology in which they etched narrow trenches into a silicon substrate, passivated the trench walls, and then etched the channel starting from the trench bottom. A conformally deposited polysilicon layer closed off the trench, followed by a front-side deep reactive ion etch (DRIE) step to define the needle shape and a back-side DRIE etch to thin the substrate; DRIE permits etching straight into a silicon substrate, forming trenches with vertical side walls. Their microneedles had a 100-µm-wide, 100-µm-thick, and 2-mm-long shaft with a microchannel diameter of 20 µm. Lee et al. (3) developed a fabrication technology based on a combination of DRIE vertically into silicon and glass bonding and reflow to provide a channel cover. They formed microneedles up to 5.3 mm in length and 70 µm wide and 40 µm in thickness. These extremely slender and long microneedles were intended for precise fluid injection into brain tissue. Lee et al. (4) developed a fabrication process for micromachining microdialysis probes. A length of 4 mm of their 180-µm-wide and 45-µm-thick silicon probe was covered with a 5-µm-thick polysilicon membrane with 60–80-nm-wide straight pores etched into it. The probe contained a 30-µm-deep and 60-µm-wide U-shaped channel.

Other approaches based on surface micromachining were developed by Brazzle et al. (5) and Takeuchi et al. (6), both forming needle structures around sacrificial photoresist. Brazzle et al. used electroforming of nickel to fabricate microneedles on sacrificial photoresist layers patterned on a silicon membrane. The microneedle structures were 2 mm long with an inner channel of approximately 30 µm in width and 20 µm in height, and outer dimensions of approximately 80 µm in width and 60 µm in height. Fabrication of polymer in-plane microneedle neural probes was demonstrated by Takeuchi et al. A flexible needle-like probe was formed by deposition of parylene beneath and on top of a sacrificial photoresist layer corresponding to the inner channel. The resulting probes were several millimeters long with 200-µm-wide inner channels. As the high flexibility of the parylene structure did not allow penetration into the tissue, the authors proposed filling the needle channels with polyethylene glycol (PEG) temporarily prior to tissue penetration, to improve its rigidity. Stupar and Pisano (7) formed similar parylene microneedles around sacrificial silicon. The outline of a microneedle structure was first patterned, in the in-plane direction, through a thin silicon wafer using DRIE. A thick parylene layer was then vapor-deposited as the structural layer. The sacrificial silicon was then etched using KOH to create the hollow parylene microneedles. By partially etching the silicon, stiffer microneedles were made containing parylene shafts and single-crystal silicon tips. The resulting microneedles were able to endure very large deflection angles of up to 180°. A 2.65-mm-long microneedle with a width of 240 µm and wall thickness of 20 µm was measured to have a bending stiffness of 63.5 N/m.

Lippmann et al. (8) demonstrated a different approach for manufacturing polymeric microneedles involving a combination of injection molding and investment casting performed at micron scale. After placement of investment wires into silicon micromachined inserts, the inserts were put into an injection mold assembly. Polymer was then injected into the insert cavity to create needle-like structures. After releasing the molded structures from the assembly, the hollow core of the needles was formed by dissolving the investment wires. Using this process, needles with rectangular cross-sections of 130 µm × 100 µm were created with lengths of 280 µm and an inner diameter of 35 µm. Tapered needles were also created with triangular cross-sections, with two sides of 105 µm in width and one of 150 µm; they had a base-to-tip length of 300 µm and the same inner diameter of 35 µm.

Talbot and Pisano (9) and Zahn et al. (10) developed a molding technique for polysilicon microneedles. They etched a mold straight into a silicon wafer using DRIE. Through holes were etched from the backside using KOH. They then deposited phosphosilicate glass onto this wafer and onto a blank silicon wafer. Both wafers were pressure-bonded together at 1000°C. During the deposition of 15–20 µm of polysilicon, the polysilicon entered the mold by the through holes and deposited on the inside wall of the mold and on the outside. After removal of the polysilicon from the outside using reactive ion etching, a release etch in concentrated hydrofluoric acid removed the phosphosilicate glass, separated the two mold wafers, and freed the polysilicon needle structures from the mold. The needles had a thickness of 110 µm, a width of 160 µm, a wall thickness of 15–20 µm, and a typical length of 4.5 mm.

4.2.2 Out-of-Plane Microneedles

Out-of-plane microneedles with their shafts perpendicular to the base substrate plane allow for two-dimensional arrangements; they can therefore cover a larger tissue area than in-plane microneedle designs, which can be advantageous for particular applications. Out-of-plane microneedles are in general formed either through subtractive manufacturing such as bulk micromachining of silicon or through additive manufacturing including thin film processing and molding of metals, polymers, ceramics, or polycrystalline silicon. In subtractive manufacturing, the needle lumen is etched into the substrate; in additive manufacturing, the hollow core emerges as material is deposited around a temporary core structure.

4.2.2.1 Silicon Out-of-Plane Microneedles

Fabrication methods for hollow silicon microneedles have first been presented in 2000 (11), not long after DRIE was introduced as a new micromachining process. DRIE permits etching straight into silicon, enabling the formation of channels through a silicon wafer that can form the inner lumens of microneedles; the outer shape of these needles can be achieved through a variety of etching processes that remove the silicon such that only the silicon forming the needles remains along with a backing plate connecting the needles of an array. Figure 4.1 shows schematics of representative fabrication processes for hollow silicon microneedles. In all cases, the needle lumen is formed using DRIE before machining the outer

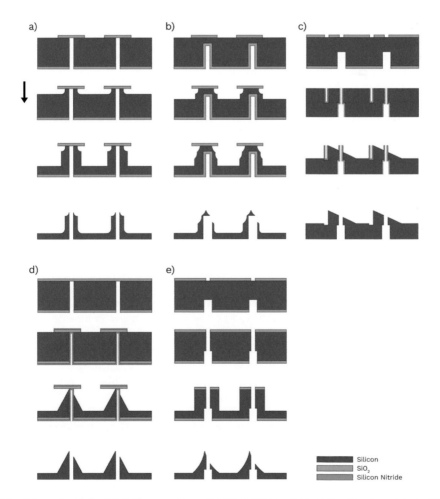

FIGURE 4.1 Schematic of the fabrication processes of hollow silicon microneedles, based on data in **(a)** ref. (13), **(b)** ref. (14), **(c)** ref. (16), **(d)** ref. (17), and **(e)** ref. (18).

shape of the needles. The needle shape can be created through a combination of isotropic dry etching and DRIE as shown in Figure 4.1a (12, 13) and Figure 4.1b (14, 15); through anisotropic etching taking advantage of the crystalline structure of silicon as shown in Figure 4.1c (16) and 4.1d (17); or through a dicing saw followed by a wet etching process as shown in Figure 4.1e (18).

All the silicon out-of-plane microneedle designs offer the possibility of a side opening where a sharp needle tip initiates penetration into the target tissue. In addition, the design by Griss and Stemme (14) positions the tip above the lumen with lumen openings on rather vertical areas of the needle shaft. This design, which extends the needle length significantly, was intended to prevent coring – that is, the creation of a tissue plug during insertion, thought to be an issue in other designs.

4.2.2.2 Polymer Out-of-Plane Microneedles

Polymers are attractive materials for microneedle fabrication due to their low material and processing cost. However, their lower strength compared to silicon and metals imposes limitations on the needle size. To achieve a strength comparable to that of metal or silicon microneedles, polymer microneedles require a much greater wall thickness, which often results in devices substantially larger and with a smaller aspect ratio than other microneedle types.

Plastic injection molding has also been used to manufacture polymer microneedles. The limitations of computer numerical control (CNC) machining in creating high-aspect-ratio cavities, and the difficulties of injecting molten plastic through narrow cavities without degradation, lead to constraints on the size of the manufactured needles.

An example of the result of plastic injection molding is presented by Yung et al. (19). These microneedles have lengths of 500 µm and tip diameters of 110 µm. However, despite performance of a preliminary penetration experiment into pig skin samples, sufficient strength of these structures has not been demonstrated in clinical applications or through bench testing. The Hollow Microstructured Transdermal System (hMTS) by 3M (St. Paul, MN, US) is another example of an injection-molded microneedle device consisting of arrays of 500–900 µm microstructures with 10–40 µm lumen diameters.

Other methods for fabricating polymer microneedles have been proposed. Moon et al. (20, 21) used a process involving two successive inclined photoresist exposure steps to fabricate polymer tetrahedral-shaped microneedles with heights in the range 750–1000 µm and lumen diameters of 190–400 µm. The resulting devices have sharp tips but are limited in aspect ratio and array spacing. Huang and Fu (22) proposed a process for making polymer microneedles involving a patterned polydimethylsiloxane (PDMS) base layer on a patterned glass assembly, followed by forming needle structures on the PDMS layer from photo-patternable SU-8 epoxy through photolithography. The resulting needles were 200 µm high; however, their mechanical strength for reliable skin penetration has not been demonstrated.

A scalable method for producing polymer microneedles presented by Mansoor et al. (23) is shown in Figure 4.2. This method involves deposition of a thin polydimethylsiloxane (PDMS) layer onto a mold containing a number of vertical posts, followed by deposition of the microneedle structural polymer layer using solvent casting. Prior to the casting of the microneedle structural layer, a plasma treatment step was used to ensure better wetting and adhesion of the microneedle structural layer to the PDMS substrate. Separation of the array was performed by mechanical force. Opening of the tips was achieved by a plasma etching step prior to separation from the mold, which removed the structural polymer from the tip because the structural layer is thin in that region.

Using this process, polyimide microneedles with 2 wt% clay reinforcement were fabricated. The needles were 280 µm tall, and had tip and base diameters of 65 µm and 115 µm, respectively. The strength of the structures was evaluated under axial compressive loading with a failure load of about 0.17 N.

Another example of a ceramic-reinforced polymer microneedle was presented by Ovsianikov et al. (24) who used an optical two-photon polymerization system to manufacture 3D cross-linked structures from an organically modified ceramic hybrid material (Ormocer®). Hollow microneedles with 800 µm height and base diameters in the range 150–300 µm were manufactured. The resulting devices were shown to be capable of puncturing porcine adipose tissue.

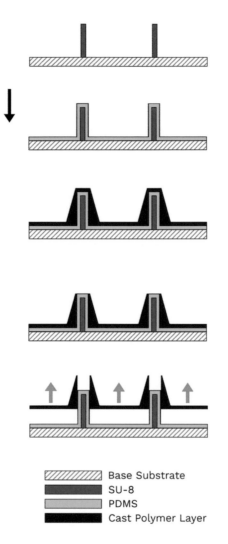

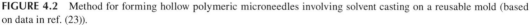

FIGURE 4.2 Method for forming hollow polymeric microneedles involving solvent casting on a reusable mold (based on data in ref. (23)).

4.2.2.3 Metal Out-of-Plane Microneedles

Hollow metallic microneedles offer several advantages over silicon or polymeric microneedles in terms of fabrication costs and mechanical strength. The most common fabrication technique involves electro-deposition of metal onto a mold that is later either removed through etching or dissolving in a solvent or separated from the metallic layer.

Figure 4.3 shows some reported MEMS-based fabrication processes that commonly involve creating cone-shaped high-aspect-ratio post structures extending from a planar surface, and then using them as template for subsequent metal electrodeposition. In these processes, the length and diameter of the post structures control the needle length and lumen size, respectively. The duration of the electrodeposition step determines the thickness of the structural metal layer, which impacts robustness of the needle shaft. Several such processes for metal microneedles made using electrodeposition have been developed that differ in their approach to create the conductive seed layer required for electroplating, the method used to separate the microneedles from the template, and the method for achieving open needle tips. These processes allow microneedles to be manufactured in a wide range of dimensions. Outer diameters ranging from 30 μm to 125 μm (at the tip) and lengths ranging from 200 μm to 1800 μm have been reported.

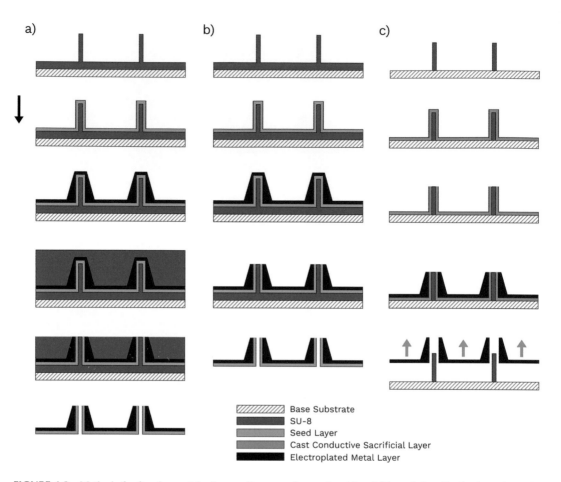

FIGURE 4.3 Methods for forming metal microneedles around posts that **(a)** and **(b)** are being dissolved to release the needles or **(c)** can be reused for subsequent fabrication processes (**a**, based on data from ref. (25); **b**, based on data from refs (26 and 27); **c**, based on data from ref. (29)).

After creating template structures from the negative photoresist SU-8 using photolithography, Kim et al. (25) deposited a Cr-Cu seed metal layer using sputter deposition followed by electroplating of the structural nickel layer (Figure 4.3a). Next, another SU-8 layer was added that embedded the metal layer. This temporary support structure facilitated mechanical polishing of the microneedle tips to open them up. Finally, dry etching of the SU-8 layers was achieved using O_2/CF_4 plasma, yielding arrays of hollow metal microneedles. Li et al. (26) used SU-8 drawing lithography to create tall mold structures (Figure 4.3b). After depositing a silver seed layer, nickel was electroplated to form microneedles. The tip of the microneedle was removed through laser cutting, followed by dissolving the SU-8 template in a liquid solvent. Lee et al. (27) used a similar method, but instead of laser cutting the tips, they used a non-conductive masking layer to coat the top of the conductive seed layer prior to plating, to prevent metal electroplating in this area and to ensure that the tips of the final device are open. Another method by Kobayashi and Suzuki (28) created a microneedle by plating on a conductive wire protruding from a base substrate, and the opened tip of the microneedle was achieved by adding a protective mask to the tip of the wire prior to plating; the wire was then dissolved leaving the plated metal shell as the needle structure. Another approach, shown in Figure 4.3c, by Mansoor et al. (29) used solvent casting to coat an array of SU-8 pillars with a polymer-based conductive sacrificial layer. A plasma etching step was then used to selectively etch the solvent cast coating covering the tip of the SU-8 pillars. After electroplating nickel onto the conductive coating, the microneedle array was separated by dissolving the conductive coating. The SU-8 mold could then be reused for repeated manufacturing of microneedles.

Norman et al. (30) used multiple replica molding steps to create sacrificial replicas of a master mold containing a cone-shaped pillar structure with a laser-ablated cavity at the tip. After sputtering a seed layer onto the sacrificial molds, metal was electrodeposited to form microneedles. As the metal did not coat the deep cavities at the tip, the resulting structures were open at the tip. Microneedles with inner tip diameters of 20 μm and lengths of 1100 μm were fabricated with this method.

Using silicon as sacrificial substrate in metal microneedle fabrication was demonstrated by McAllister et al. (31) and Shikida et al. (32). Shikida et al. fabricated silicon structures with hourglass-like shapes by a combination of dicing and anisotropic etching steps. Next a Cr-Au seed layer was deposited on the structures. During this step, the top surface of the hourglass-shaped structures acted as shadow mask preventing metal deposition on side walls of the upper portion of the structures. Nickel was then electroplated to fabricate the microneedle structural layer, and the silicon etched away using anisotropic etching. Microneedles of various tip-opening shapes were made with heights ranging from 120 μm to 250 μm.

A number of previous studies have formed metallic microneedles on negative molds containing a cavity on which metal is plated. An overview of such a process is shown in Figure 4.4. McAllister et al. (31) used solid silicon microneedles (formed by anisotropic SF_6/O_2 plasma etching of silicon) as a master to form metallic microneedles using a polymeric mold. After deposition of SU-8 epoxy on the silicon structures, a plasma etching step was used to expose their tips. The silicon structures were then selectively removed by SF_6 plasma or HNO_3/HF solution, leaving an SU-8 epoxy mold as a negative of the microneedles. After deposition of a seed layer, a NiFe layer was deposited onto the mold to form microneedles. Arrays of 20×20 were made with 150 μm spacing. The needles were 150 μm in height with a base diameter of 80 μm and a tip diameter of 10 μm. Davis et al. (33) drilled holes through a polymer substrate using a laser. The substrate was then coated by a conductive seed layer followed by electroplating of a nickel layer to form the needles. Next, the polymer substrate was selectively etched leaving the microneedles behind. As the laser-drilled holes were through holes, the resulting devices were open at the tip. Microneedles with heights of 50–1000 μm and diameters of 50–400 μm have been manufactured.

Examples of metallic microneedles made through conventional machining techniques have also been reported (i.e., Micropoint Technologies Hollow Microneedle Hub or Becton Dickinson Soluvia

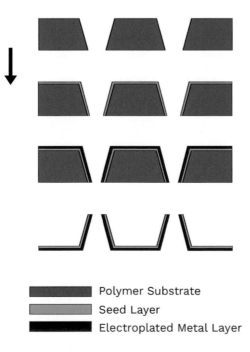

Polymer Substrate
Seed Layer
Electroplated Metal Layer

FIGURE 4.4 Formation of metal microneedles by metal electrodeposition onto the surface of a laser-drilled through hole.

Microinjection System). Machined microneedles are large in size due to the limitations of the conventional machining tools. The typical lengths are 1–1.5 mm with diameters comparable to those of conventional 31 or 32G hypodermic needles. Due to these lengths, liquid injection occurs in deeper skin layers or in subcutaneous tissue.

4.2.2.4 Silica and Ceramic Microneedles

Similar to silicon microneedles, devices made from silicon dioxide (SiO_2) or ceramics are brittle and thus prone to fracture inside the skin during application.

One common manufacturing method for SiO_2 microneedles uses a combination of etching into the bulk of the silicon substrate followed by a thermal oxidation step to grow a silicon dioxide layer that will later form the needle upon subsequent etching of the initial silicon mold. The same process limitations as for silicon needles also apply to SiO_2 needles. In addition, the SiO_2 needles are much more brittle than silicon needles since the thickness of the oxide layer is limited resulting in fragile structures. Khanna et al. (34) used masking steps and DRIE to create deep channels, which were later coated with SiO_2 through thermal oxidation. Similarly, through a combination of DRIE and selective vapor-liquid-solid growth, Takei et al. (35) created a mold for subsequent SiO_2 deposition. Another process presented by Rodriguez et al. (36) used a similar approach involving multiple silicon substrate etching steps using tetramethylammonium hydroxide (TMAH) to create deep high-aspect-ratio channels. After growing an oxide layer on the channel surfaces, buffered HF etching was used to partially remove the oxide layer to open the needle tips. Another approach has been presented by Rajaraman and Henderson (37) in which a coherent porous silicon (CPS) etching technology is used to fabricate deep channels that are then used to grow a structural oxide layer. Strambini et al. (38) used back-side illumination electrochemical etching (BIEE) to create deep channels in a silicon substrate on which an oxide layer was then formed. In all these techniques, a process step involves etching of a silicon substrate mold to reveal the oxide structures.

4.3 Mechanical Strength

Microneedle strength is important to avoid breakage during insertion or handling. Many microneedles have therefore been tested for buckling strength through axial loading and also for shear or bending breakage due to lateral loads.

Talbot et al. (10) applied a lateral force to their 4.5-mm-long polysilicon microneedles and observed failure at around 56 mN. The failure load almost doubled for needles that were coated with a 10-µm-thick layer of platinum or nickel. Paik et al. (2) found that their 2-mm-long silicon needles had a buckling strength of 3.06 N to 6.28 N depending on the particular shaft design, while the tapered tips broke at loads between 146 mN and 276 mN. The maximum average bending load of these needles was 124 mN. The needles were sufficiently strong for insertion into rabbit ear skin. Khanna et al. (39) determined the axial and shear fracture strength of 200-µm-tall silicon microneedles that had outer diameters from 100 µm to 200 µm with a wall thickness of 35–50 µm. The needles with 100 µm outer diameter collapsed under 7.4 N of axial load. The shear fracture strength increased from 0.36 N to 2.75 N when increasing the needle diameter from 100 µm to 200 µm. In all three cases, failure occurred near the fracture strength of silicon around 700 MPa.

Khanna et al. (34) evaluated the strength of silicon dioxide microneedles with circular and square tip shapes, formed through silicon thermal oxidation, by measuring the axial and shear fracture strength of the devices. The axial fracture strength of these microneedles was 30 mN for a circular tip and 20 mN for a square tip. The shear fracture strength of these microneedles were 22 mN for a circular tip and 6 mN for a square tip.

Mansoor et al. (23) reported a strength of 320 mN, under axial loading, for clay-reinforced polyimide microneedles formed through solvent casting. The strength was shown to be sufficient for insertion of microneedles into excised rabbit ear skin.

Li et al. (26) measured the axial fracture load of 1.8-mm microneedles made from nickel and compared that with the force required to penetrate a polyurethane skin model. The measurements were performed on microneedles with bevel angles of 15° and 90° (with respect to the axial direction). The skin penetration forces were measured to be 1.63 ± 0.07 N and 0.83 ± 0.05 N and the fracture forces 5.97 ± 0.14 N and 5.85 ± 0.25 N for 15° and 90° bevel angles, respectively. Lee et al. (27) compared axial fracture forces of nickel microneedles of different lengths. The axial load fracture force of a microneedle with 10-μm wall thickness was 1 ± 0.13 N for a 600-μm length, 0.28 ± 0.4N for a 1200-μm length, and below 0.1 N for a 1800-μm length. Increasing the wall thickness of an 1800-μm-long microneedle to 20 or 30 μm increased the fracture force to 0.34 ± 0.18 N and 3.16 ± 0.09 N, respectively. Mansoor et al. (29) measured the fracture force of 500-μm-tall nickel microneedles with tip lumen diameter of 40 μm and tip wall thickness of 15 μm to be 4.2 ± 0.61 N under axial loading. Another study by Davis et al. (40) showed a similar fracture force under axial loading for 500-μm-tall metallic nickel microneedles, and also showed that the fracture force is insensitive to tip radius for radii ranging from 40 μm to 65 μm, and the fracture force increases significantly with wall thickness from 4 μm to 15 μm and slightly with wall angle from 60° to 70°. Kim et al. (25) presented an analytical solution for critical buckling of tapered metallic nickel microneedles, indicating a high sensitivity of the critical buckling force with respect to the height of the microneedles, and showing that the critical buckling force drops as the height increases.

A direct comparison of the strength of the different microneedles is difficult because of their different geometries and dimensions. However, if one assumes that considerations for strength were included in the needle designs and the designs tested were reasonably manufacturable, one can make the following observations: polymer microneedles are the least robust. Microneedles made from brittle silicon or silicon dioxide show very low shear fracture strength and their tapered tip breaks easily under axial load. The tested silicon and nickel microneedles show a comparable axial robustness, while the tested silicon structures had mechanically more favorable dimensions. When metal needles collapse under axial load, they mainly bend without pieces breaking off, while silicon needles disintegrate. The ductility of the metal therefore reduces the possibility of pieces breaking off in the skin during application under excessive loading. As a result, they are less likely to remain partially in the tissue, which could be a concern for other materials.

4.4 Needle Integration

Integration methods of hollow microneedle arrays with secondary systems have to take the microneedle material and the intended application into consideration. In intradermal drug delivery systems, the high liquid pressures involved in intradermal injection (41) settings requires a strong seal between the microneedle arrays and the supporting structures. For silicon, due to its brittleness, the most common integration method for this application is adhesive bonding of the array to a rigid backing such as brass (14) or plastic (13, 42) that provides a support for the majority of the backing plate. In addition, there exist several direct bonding methods for silicon. The irreversible chemical bonding of plasma surface-activated PDMS and silicon has been used to bond a chip with a row of in-plane silicon needles to a PDMS channel system (2) or to generate an integrated MEMS syringe (43); however, the flexibility of PDMS and the large unsupported area above the fluid reservoir make this silicon-needle-based MEMS syringe very fragile. Anodic bonding forms an irreversible bond between silicon and Pyrex™ and has been used to integrate an array of silicon microneedles with a channel system etched into the back side of the needle backing with a Pyrex™ chip for fluid extraction (18).

Roxhed et al. (15) fabricated silicon microneedles coated with a thin (170–470 nm) layer of gold that also covered the needle opening. This seal was supposed to prevent liquid leakage before needle insertion into tissue. The 170-nm-thick gold membranes were shown to burst at a pressure of 120 kPa, by electrochemical means within 2 min, or through full needle insertion into human skin in vivo.

Rodrigues et al. (36) bonded silicon dioxide microneedles to a glass support and then by means of an epoxy connected the assembly to a flexible tube ending in a syringe. The fixture, though, was not tested under any high-pressure application to assess the strength of the bonding.

Takei et al. (35) used resin to integrate a silicon dioxide microneedle device, formed on silicon substrate, to a flexible tube connected to a syringe. The setup was then used to deliver DI water to a rat model using a pressure of about 40 kPa.

Plastic and metallic microneedles have mostly been integrated with polymer support structures using adhesives and sealing materials. For example, Mansoor et al. (23) used adhesives to bond polymeric microneedle to a plastic Luer fitting that attached to a syringe. Kobayashi et al. (28) integrated a metallic microneedle into a sampling system by using silicone rubber at the base of the microneedle structure to provide a seal.

4.5 Insertion Methods

The shape of microneedles plays a significant role in the insertion process, in particular for the required insertion force. Roxhed et al. (44) required 10 mN per needle to insert an array or 25 silicon microneedles with a sharp tip (tip radius below 100 nm) into human skin in vivo. Khanna et al. (45) used silicon microneedles that were sharpened to different degrees by reducing the width of the ring-shaped tip area. For slow insertion into skin tissue, the insertion force for a 4×4 microneedle array dropped from 4.80 N to 0.11 N when reducing the ring area per needle from 11,100 μm^2 to 186 μm^2. Davis et al. (33) determined that the average force required to insert a 500-μm-long metallic microneedle, with tip diameter of 75 μm, into human skin is approximately 0.2 N. In another work, Davis et al. (40) presents a theoretical model that describes the insertion force of the microneedles (with flat tips) as a function of the needle tip area. The model assumes a linear relationship between the insertion force and the needle tip area. Further experimental work done with microneedles of various tip areas (ranging from 2500 μm^2 to 20000 μm^2) showed results consistent with the theoretical prediction. Li et al. (26) reported that the average force required for skin penetration by 1800-μm-long metallic microneedles with bevel angles of $90°$ and $15°$ (with respect to the axial direction) was 1.63 ± 0.07 N and 0.83 ± 0.05 N, respectively; the outer diameter of the microneedles was 120 μm. Khanna et al. (34) measured the forces of penetration for silicon dioxide microneedles into cadaver human skin. An array of 15×15 needles with 1000 μm pitch penetrated the skin samples at about 20 mN. The microneedles were circular in lumen shape, with 20 μm outer diameter and 100–120 μm height. Stupar and Pisano (7) demonstrated the penetration of in-plane hollow parylene microneedles into a gelatin membrane. The force required for penetration was measured at 0.45 N, for 4.5-mm-long, 200-μm-wide needles with 50-μm wall thicknesses.

Verbaan et al. (46) produced 4×4 arrays of 300–900-μm-long needles made from commercially available 30G hypodermic needles, and showed that needles of 550 μm length or longer can be manually inserted into excised human skin, while manual insertion of 300-μm-long needles fails. Several researchers have developed insertion devices that impart a high velocity onto the needles facilitating tissue penetration. Verbaan et al. (47) applied arrays of 16–81 245-μm-long silicon microneedles made according to Gardeniers et al. (16) to excised human skin. Their electric applicator inserted the needles at 1 m/s or 3 m/s into skin while manual application resulted in only slight piercing of the skin. The depth of nanoparticles deposited following insertion was identical for 1 m/s and 3 m/s, while molecular diffusion through the insertion openings in the skin was slightly higher for the higher velocity. Van der Maaden et al. (48) used an applicator to insert microneedles, made from fused silica capillaries with an outer diameter of 375 μm, into human skin at a speed of 1 m/s. Chua et al. (49) applied arrays of about 260 silicon microneedles of 325–350-μm length to human skin at an impact velocity of 10 m/s. The array of needles that were tapered along the entire shaft at an angle of about $10°$ caused mainly mode-I cracks where the needles wedged open the cracks as they advanced. The array of more blunt needles resulted mainly in mode-II cracks where circular regions of tissue propagate ahead of the needles. They used both arrays for a glucose sensing application and noticed that the signal collected with the array of blunt needles was weaker than the signal from the more pointed needles, indicating a slight obstruction of the blunt needles related to mode-II crack formation.

4.6 Conclusions

A wide variety of hollow microneedle designs have been developed that differ in geometry, manufacturing method, and materials. Many of the manufacturing methods described in this chapter are suitable for large-scale manufacturing, while some will not go beyond lab scale. In-plane designs are particularly advantageous for integrating electrodes and flow control elements, while out-of-plane designs can be used for larger arrays, and they allow more convenient integration with large-scale flow control systems. The low rigidity of polymers makes it challenging to produce polymeric microneedles with small dimensions that are capable of penetrating the stratum corneum. Silicon, silicon dioxide, and metals are sufficiently rigid, but manufacturing silicon dioxide structures with significant wall thicknesses is challenging; both silicon and silicon dioxide are brittle and risk breaking under shear forces, and microneedles made from these materials are therefore more difficult to integrate than metal microneedles. These considerations should guide the choice of a particular design for a given application.

REFERENCES

1. Lin L, Pisano AP. Silicon-processed microneedles. J Microelectromechanical Syst. 1999 Mar;8(1):78–84.
2. Paik S-J, Byun S, Lim J-M, Park Y, Lee A, Chung S, et al. In-plane single-crystal-silicon microneedles for minimally invasive microfluid systems. Sens Actuators Phys. 2004 Sep 1;114(2):276–84.
3. Lee HJ, Son Y, Kim D, Kim YK, Choi N, Yoon E-S, et al. A new thin silicon microneedle with an embedded microchannel for deep brain drug infusion. Sens Actuators B Chem. 2015 Mar 31;209:413–22.
4. Lee WH, Ngernsutivorakul T, Mabrouk OS, Wong J-MT, Dugan CE, Pappas SS, et al. Microfabrication and in vivo performance of a microdialysis probe with embedded membrane. Anal Chem. 2016 Jan 19;88(2):1230–7.
5. Brazzle JD, Papautsky I, Frazier AB. Hollow metallic micromachined needle arrays. Biomed Microdevices. 2000 Jun 1;2(3):197–205.
6. Takeuchi S, Ziegler D, Yoshida Y, Mabuchi K, Suzuki T. Parylene flexible neural probes integrated with microfluidic channels. Lab Chip. 2005;5(5):519.
7. Stupar PA, Pisano AP. Silicon, parylene, and silicon/parylene micro-needles for strength and toughness. In: The 11th International Conference on Solid-State Sensors and Actuators. Berlin, Heidelberg; 2001. pp. 1358–61.
8. Lippmann JM, Geiger EJ, Pisano AP. Polymer investment molding: Method for fabricating hollow, microscale parts. Sens Actuators Phys. 2007 Feb 28;134(1):2–10.
9. Talbot NH, Pisano AP. Polymolding: Two wafer polysilicon micromolding of closed-flow passages for microneedles and microfluidic devices. In: 1998 Solid State Sensor and Actuator Workshop. Hilton Head, S.C.; 1998. pp. 265–8.
10. Zahn JD, Talbot NH, Liepmann D, Pisano AP. Microfabricated polysilicon microneedles for minimally invasive biomedical devices. Biomed Microdevices. 2000 Dec 1;2(4):295–303.
11. Stoeber B, Liepmann D. Fluid injection through out-of-plane microneedles. In: 1st Annual International IEEE-EMBS Special Topic Conference on Microtechnologies in Medicine and Biology Proceedings (Cat No00EX451). 2000. pp. 224–8.
12. Zimmermann S, Fienbork D, Stoeber B, Flounders AW, Liepmann D. A microneedle-based glucose monitor: Fabricated on a wafer-level using in-device enzyme immobilization. In: TRANSDUCERS, Solid-State Sensors, Actuators and Microsystems, 12th International Conference on, 2003. 2003. pp. 99–102 vol.1.
13. Stoeber B, Liepmann D. Arrays of hollow out-of-plane microneedles for drug delivery. J Microelectromechanical Syst. 2005 Jun;14(3):472–9.
14. Griss P, Stemme G. Side-opened out-of-plane microneedles for microfluidic transdermal liquid transfer. J Microelectromechanical Syst. 2003 Jun;12(3):296–301.
15. Roxhed N, Griss P, Stemme G. Membrane-sealed hollow microneedles and related administration schemes for transdermal drug delivery. Biomed Microdevices. 2008 Apr;10(2):271–9.
16. Gardeniers HJGE, Luttge R, Berenschot EJW, Boer MJ de, Yeshurun SY, Hefetz M, et al. Silicon micromachined hollow microneedles for transdermal liquid transport. J Microelectromechanical Syst. 2003 Dec;12(6):855–62.
17. Jurcicek P, Zou H, Zhang S, Liu C. Design and fabrication of hollow out-of-plane silicon microneedles. IET Micro Nano Lett. 2013 Feb;8(2):78–81.
18. Mukerjee EV, Collins SD, Isseroff RR, Smith RL. Microneedle array for transdermal biological fluid extraction and in situ analysis. Sens Actuators Phys. 2004 Sep 1;114(2):267–75.
19. Yung KL, Xu Y, Kang C, Liu H, Tam KF, Ko SM, et al. Sharp tipped plastic hollow microneedle array by microinjection moulding. J Micromechanics Microengineering. 2012 Jan 1;22(1):015016.

20. Moon SJ, Lee SS, Lee HS, Kwon TH. Fabrication of microneedle array using LIGA and hot embossing process. Microsyst Technol. 2005 Apr 1;11(4–5):311–8.
21. Moon SJ, Lee SS. A novel fabrication method of a microneedle array using inclined deep x-ray exposure. J Micromechanics Microengineering. 2005;15(5):903.
22. Huang H, Fu C. Different fabrication methods of out-of-plane polymer hollow needle arrays and their variations. J Micromechanics Microengineering. 2007 Feb 1;17(2):393–402.
23. Mansoor I, Hafeli UO, Stoeber B. Hollow out-of-plane polymer microneedles made by solvent casting for transdermal drug delivery. J Microelectromechanical Syst. 2012 Feb;21(1):44–52.
24. Ovsianikov A, Chichkov B, Mente P, Monteiro-Riviere NA, Doraiswamy A, Narayan RJ. Two photon polymerization of polymer-ceramic hybrid materials for transdermal drug delivery. Int J Appl Ceram Technol. 2007 Jan;4(1):22–9.
25. Kim K, Park DS, Lu HM, Che W, Kim K, Lee J-B, et al. A tapered hollow metallic microneedle array using backside exposure of SU-8. J Micromechanics Microengineering. 2004 Apr 1;14(4):597–603.
26. Li CG, Lee CY, Lee K, Jung H. An optimized hollow microneedle for minimally invasive blood extraction. Biomed Microdevices. 2013 Feb;15(1):17–25.
27. Lee K, Lee HC, Lee D-S, Jung H. Drawing lithography: Three-dimensional fabrication of an ultrahigh-aspect-ratio microneedle. Adv Mater. 2010 Jan 26;22(4):483–6.
28. Kobayashi K, Suzuki H. A sampling mechanism employing the phase transition of a gel and its application to a micro analysis system imitating a mosquito. Sens Actuators B Chem. 2001 Nov 1;80(1):1–8.
29. Mansoor I, Liu Y, Häfeli UO, Stoeber B. Arrays of hollow out-of-plane microneedles made by metal electrodeposition onto solvent cast conductive polymer structures. J Micromechanics Microengineering. 2013;23(8):085011.
30. Norman JJ, Choi S-O, Tong NT, Aiyar AR, Patel SR, Prausnitz MR, et al. Hollow microneedles for intradermal injection fabricated by sacrificial micromolding and selective electrodeposition. Biomed Microdevices. 2013 Apr;15(2):203–10.
31. McAllister D, Cros F, Davis S, Matta L, Prausnitz M, Allen M. Three-dimensional hollow microneedle and microtube arrays, Technical Digest of Transducers'99, International Conference on Solid-State Sensors and Actuators, Sendai, 1999 June 7-10, pp 1098–1101.
32. Shikida M, Hasada T, Sato K. Fabrication of a hollow needle structure by dicing, wet etching and metal deposition. J Micromechanics Microengineering. 2006;16(10):2230.
33. Davis SP, Martanto W, Allen MG, Prausnitz MR. Hollow metal microneedles for insulin delivery to diabetic rats. IEEE Trans Biomed Eng. 2005 May;52(5):909–15.
34. Khanna P, Flam BR, Osborn B, Strom JA, Bhansali S. Skin penetration and fracture strength testing of silicon dioxide microneedles. Sens Actuators Phys. 2011 Nov 1;170(1):180–6.
35. Takei K, Kawashima T, Kawano T, Kaneko H, Sawada K, Ishida M. Out-of-plane microtube arrays for drug delivery—liquid flow properties and an application to the nerve block test. Biomed Microdevices. 2009 Jun 1;11(3):539–45.
36. Rodriguez A, Molinero D, Valera E, Trifonov T, Marsal LF, Pallarès J, et al. Fabrication of silicon oxide microneedles from macroporous silicon. Sens Actuators B Chem. 2005 Aug 24;109(1):135–40.
37. Rajaraman S, Henderson HT. A unique fabrication approach for microneedles using coherent porous silicon technology. Sens Actuators B Chem. 2005 Mar 28;105(2):443–8.
38. Strambini LM, Longo A, Diligenti A, Barillaro G. A minimally invasive microchip for transdermal injection/sampling applications. Lab Chip. 2012 Aug 14;12(18):3370–9.
39. Khanna P, Luongo K, Strom JA, Bhansali S. Axial and shear fracture strength evaluation of silicon microneedles. Microsyst Technol. 2010 Jun 1;16(6):973–8.
40. Davis SP, Landis BJ, Adams ZH, Allen MG, Prausnitz MR. Insertion of microneedles into skin: measurement and prediction of insertion force and needle fracture force. J Biomech. 2004 Aug;37(8):1155–63.
41. Gupta J, Park SS, Bondy B, Felner EI, Prausnitz MR. Infusion pressure and pain during microneedle injection into skin of human subjects. Biomaterials. 2011 Oct;32(28):6823–31.
42. Van Damme P, Oosterhuis-Kafeja F, Van der Wielen M, Almagor Y, Sharon O, Levin Y. Safety and efficacy of a novel microneedle device for dose sparing intradermal influenza vaccination in healthy adults. Vaccine. 2009 Jan 14;27(3):454–9.
43. Häfeli UO, Mokhtari A, Liepmann D, Stoeber B. In vivo evaluation of a microneedle-based miniature syringe for intradermal drug delivery. Biomed Microdevices. 2009 Oct;11(5):943–50.

44. Roxhed N, Gasser TC, Griss P, Holzapfel GA, Stemme G. Penetration-enhanced ultrasharp microneedles and prediction on skin interaction for efficient transdermal drug delivery. J Microelectromechanical Syst. 2007 Dec;16(6):1429–40.
45. Khanna P, Luongo K, Strom JA, Bhansali S. Sharpening of hollow silicon microneedles to reduce skin penetration force. J Micromechanics Microengineering. 2010;20(4):045011.
46. Verbaan FJ, Bal SM, van den Berg DJ, Groenink WHH, Verpoorten H, Lüttge R, et al. Assembled microneedle arrays enhance the transport of compounds varying over a large range of molecular weight across human dermatomed skin. J Control Release Off J Control Release Soc. 2007 Feb 12;117(2):238–45.
47. Verbaan FJ, Bal SM, van den Berg DJ, Dijksman JA, van Hecke M, Verpoorten H, et al. Improved piercing of microneedle arrays in dermatomed human skin by an impact insertion method. J Control Release Off J Control Release Soc. 2008 May 22;128(1):80–8.
48. van der Maaden K, Trietsch SJ, Kraan H, Varypataki EM, Romeijn S, Zwier R, et al. Novel hollow microneedle technology for depth-controlled microinjection-mediated dermal vaccination: A study with polio vaccine in rats. Pharm Res. 2014 Jan 28;31:1846–54.
49. Chua B, Desai SP, Tierney MJ, Tamada JA, Jina AN. Effect of microneedles shape on skin penetration and minimally invasive continuous glucose monitoring in vivo. Sens Actuators Phys. 2013 Dec 1;203:373–81.

5

Microneedles vs. Other Transdermal Technologies

Yeakuty Jhanker
James H.N. Tran
Heather A.E. Benson
School of Pharmacy and Biomedical Sciences, Curtin Health Innovation Research Institute, Curtin University

Tarl W. Prow
Biomaterials Engineering and Nanomedicine Strand, Future Industries Institute, University of South Australia

5.1 Background

The stratum corneum (SC) is the primary physical barrier to overcome the delivery of active molecules to therapeutic sites in the skin or underlying tissues, or via the cutaneous circulation for systemic delivery. The anatomical structure and barrier properties of the skin have been reviewed in Chapter 1. To successfully achieve transdermal or intracutaneous delivery, the SC barrier must be overcome by either mechanical or chemical intervention. The focus of the preceding chapters has been the application of microneedles in a range of fabrications that can overcome the SC barrier. Here we review other approaches and technologies that have been applied to SC barrier disruption and how they compare to microneedles (Figure 5.1). Enhancement techniques include vehicle modification to include chemicals capable of enhancing solute solubility in the SC and directly disordering the SC lipid domains, and nano and microemulsion and vesicle formulations. Indirect physical methods involving the application of electrical, acoustic, laser, and magnetic energy have advanced through experimental evaluation to commercial development. Most similar to microneedles are the alternative direct penetration methods including microdermabrasion, biolistic technologies, thermal and laser ablation, and elongated microparticles (EMPs). While formulation-based modification is an important SC permeation enhancement approach, it is the indirect and direct physical enhancement methods that are most closely comparable to microneedles and are therefore the focus of this chapter. However, vehicle/formulation-based approaches are particularly relevant in considering their potential to enhance delivery in combination with microneedles, both to enhance diffusivity of solutes within microneedle-generated pores and following microneedle-based deposition in the cutaneous tissues, and in considering controlled release to optimize therapeutic outcomes following microneedle-based deposition in the skin. Recent publications utilizing microneedles incorporating smart delivery technologies to generate combined diagnostic and treatment patches for diabetes highlight the potential role of this approach in future health care (1, 2). This combination of microneedles with other delivery technologies offers new therapeutic opportunities, and is reviewed in Chapter 6.

5.2 Indirect Physical Methods

Indirect physical methods involve the application of an energy source to the skin surface to increase diffusivity of an applied solute in the SC. A variety of different energies have been investigated including electric (iontophoresis and electroporation), magnetic (magnetophoresis), acoustic (sonophoresis), and laser.

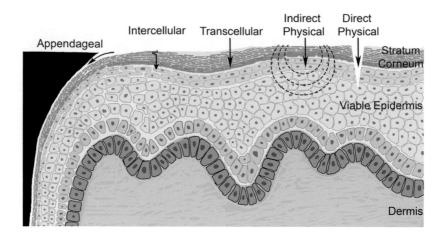

FIGURE 5.1 Routes of penetration of an API applied topically to the skin surface (appendages including hair follicles and sweat glands; intercellular and transcellular routes through the SC). Delivery enhancement approaches applied to human skin categorized as indirect and direct physical methods to enhance transport through the SC barrier.

5.2.1 Iontophoresis

In iontophoresis (Figure 5.2), a mild electric current (typically 0.1 to 1.0 mA/cm^2) is applied to increase skin permeation by three mechanisms: electromigration (the ordered movement of ions within an applied electric field as described by Faraday's law), electroosmosis (convective solvent flow in the anode-to-cathode direction due to the isoelectric point pI of 4–4.5 and negative charge of the skin), and enhanced passive diffusion (relatively minor role) (3–5). Uncharged molecules can also be delivered by these mechanisms but flux enhancement is low relative to charged molecules. The intensity of the applied current, duration of current application, and skin surface area in contact with the electrode determine iontophoretic molecular transport.

Iontophoresis has been extensively investigated for the delivery of small molecules, peptides, and proteins, and many review articles have been published (3, 6–8). A number of factors can influence iontophoretic skin delivery including: the current density and continuous/pulsed waveform, drug

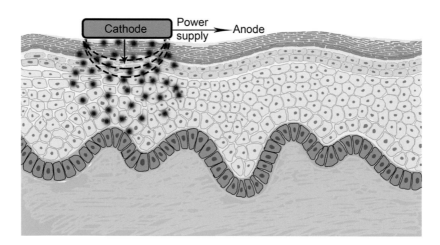

FIGURE 5.2 Iontophoretic drug delivery: a powered device consisting of an anode and a cathode generates a weak current that repels a charged solute into the skin.

concentration, vehicle pH (the degree of drug ionization affects mobility and electromigration; the degree of skin ionization determines the electroosmotic solvent flow) and molecular factors (charge/ molecular mass ratio; and volume, shape, and charge distribution of the molecule) (6). In clinical use, iontophoresis is generally well tolerated, particularly when applied as a pulsed current profile that can allow time for the skin to depolarize and return to its resting state prior to initiation of the next pulse.

A number of transdermal iontophoretic products have received regulatory approval including the LidoSite™ Topical System (lidocaine and epinephrine for local anaesthesia; Vyteris Inc., Fairlawn, NJ, USA) and Ionsys™ (fentanyl iontophoretic transdermal system for patient-controlled analgesia; developed by Alza Corporation, then acquired in sequence by Johnson & Johnson, Incline Therapeutics, and The Medicines Company and subsequently discontinued in 2017).

5.2.2 Electroporation

Electroporation involves the application of high-voltage (50–1500 V) electrical pulses lasting 10 μs to 10 ms, to generate transitory pores in the SC lipid bilayers through which applied compounds can diffuse (9). Electroporation has been shown to enhance the skin penetration of a range of molecules (9–15) but is reported to cause pain and muscle contraction (16).

5.2.3 Magnetophoresis

Magnetophoresis is the enhancement of drug permeation by the application of a magnetic field (17), 5-amino levulinic acid (18–20). Diamagnetic repulsion of the molecule into the skin is the suggested mechanism of action, although there is also some evidence of potential transient SC barrier reduction (19). We have shown that pulsed electromagnetic fields (PEMF) increased the permeation of naltrexone hydrochloride across human epidermis by 6.5× compared to passive administration (19). Gold-nanoparticle (10 nm)-treated human skin exposed to a PEMF had 200 times more gold-nanoparticle-positive pixels when visualized by multiphoton microscopy–fluorescence lifetime imaging microscopy (MPM-FLIM) than skin exposed to gold nanoparticles without PEMF. This suggests that the PEMF facilitates penetration of the gold nanoparticles through the SC and that the channels through which the nanoparticles move must be larger than 10 nm in diameter. An alternative magnetophoresis fabrication has been developed as a thin flexible polymer matrix containing multiple magnetic elements arranged to produce complex three-dimensional (3D) magnetic gradients (40 mT peak magnetic field strength; 2 T/m^2 total magnetic gradient; OBJ Ltd., Perth, Australia). This magnetic array effectively enhances flow into microneedle-porated skin to provide a synergistic permeation enhancement (21). The first commercially available magnetophoresis-based enhancer consists of the magnetic array housed in a "wand" that is used to enhance skin care products (Procter & Gamble, Cincinnati, OH).

5.2.4 Sonophoresis

Sonophoresis (phonophoresis) is the application of acoustic waves to facilitate transdermal delivery (22, 23). The main ultrasonic effects are cavitation (formation and oscillation of microbubbles; Fig. 5.3[b]), acoustic streaming, thermal effects, and direct ultrasound pressure effects on the SC bilayers. Polat et al. proposed that a microjet formed by collapse of the cavitation bubbles in the application medium generates shock waves in the SC, perturbing the barrier and increasing permeability (22). A further proposal is that the applied ultrasonic pressure waves oscillate between compression and rarefaction, transiently interrupting the continuity of the SC lipid bilayers to form pores through which applied drugs can diffuse (24).

Low-frequency ultrasound (20–100 kHz) is reported to enhance permeation of a range of molecules including macromolecules such as insulin, interferon-γ, and erythropoietin (5.8, 17, and 48 kDa respectively) across human skin in vitro (25). As low-frequency ultrasound can itself elicit

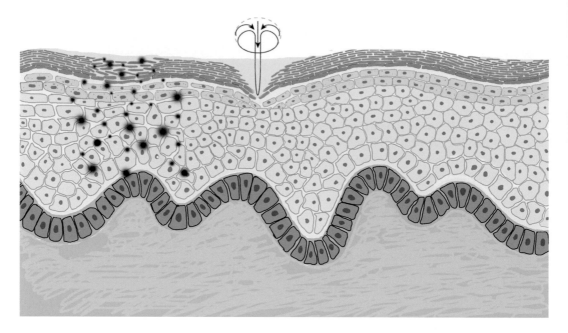

FIGURE 5.3 Sonophoresis delivery. Two proposed mechanisms of delivery: **(a)** rapid formation and oscilliation of micro-bubbles (cavitation) resulting in disruption and deformation of cells; **(b)** sonically generated microbubbles that rapidly collapse resulting in a microjet that leads to shockwave-induced cell disruption.

an immune response and activate Langerhans cells of the viable epidermis, it can act as an immunization adjuvant when coupled with a vaccine. Sonophoretic delivery of tetanus toxoid was reported to provide equal protection as an intramuscular injection when administered to mice (26, 27). Commercialized sonophoresis devices are bulky (e.g., Sonoprep®; Sontra Medical) but attempts have been made to develop wearable sonophoretic devices (28–30). A recent development is the dual administration of low and high ultrasound frequencies to increase the cavitation effect and thus skin permeability (31, 32). Schoellhammer et al. reported that a 4-min pretreatment with dual ultrasound frequencies of 20 kHz and 1 MHz, in combination with 1% SLS, enhanced the permeation of inulin and glucose across porcine skin by 3.81-fold and 13.6-fold respectively, compared to single-frequency sonophoresis (31).

5.2.5 Laser-Assisted Delivery

A photomechanical wave is generated by laser ablation of a target medium consisting of a polymer (e.g., black polystyrene) placed on the surface of the skin (33–35). The medium undergoes rapid phase change (e.g., degradation or plasma formation) resulting in the production of a shockwave through the skin below, (Figure 5.4) (36). Unlike with sonophoresis that oscillates between positive and negative pressure, no cavitation is observed. The photomechanical wave is a unipolar compressive one that disrupts the lipid arrangement within the SC intracellular space and also the cellular membranes.

In one of the earliest reports, Lee and colleagues utilized a single photomechanical wave for the delivery of nanoparticles in rats. A photomechanical wave, generated via Q-switched ruby laser ablation of black polystyrene resulting in a calculated peak pressure in the skin of 592 ± 23 bar, delivered 40 kDa rhodamine dextran to a 50 μm depth in the skin (37), and the skin remained permeable for a period after application that varied with drug size and molecular charge (2 and 40 min for 40 kDa rhodamine and amino levulinic acid, respectively) (33, 38). They also reported a 3.4-fold increase in 20-nm latex nanoparticle delivery compared to topical alone. Substantial enhancement of skin

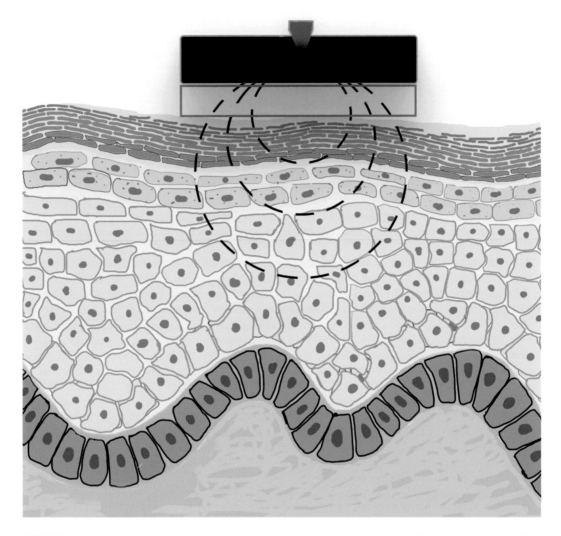

FIGURE 5.4 Laser-assisted drug delivery via photomechanical enhancement: laser is applied to a target medium (black rubber or polystyrene) situated on a reservoir containing the active compound in solution. Rapid phase change in the rubber generates shockwaves through the solution into the skin, disrupting the stratum corneum lipids and facilitating diffusion of the active compound.

delivery has been reported for a range of compounds and nanoparticles in small-animal models (34, 35, 39). Laser-generated photomechanical waves do not produce the same degree of delivery enhancement as laser-based techniques that cause ablation of the SC, as is shown by a comparative study of aminoleculinic acid with 7-, 41-, and 641-fold delivery with laser-generated photomechanical wave < fractional ablation < full ablation. The technique has received limited further interest with few publications in recent years.

5.3 Direct Physical Methods

Microneedles and their various fabrications and applications have been discussed in detail in previous chapters. While the fabrications vary from the so-called "poke and patch" to the inclusion of their medication on the surface or within the projections, they have in common the mechanism of poking an array of small, sharp projections into the skin to breach the SC barrier. Accordingly they are classified as direct physical enhancement methods. The following section reviews other technologies that are based on direct physical enhancement and thus most similar to microneedles in their enhancement mechanism.

5.3.1 Microdermabrasion

Microdermabrasion was initially developed as a technique for skin rejuvenation via superficial disruption of the skin as is utilized in dermatological and cosmeceutical practices (40, 41). This can be accomplished by instruments consisting of air-propelled particles that "sandblast" and simultaneously remove the skin by vacuum. Simple "sandpaper" approaches that are less controlled, removing larger/deeper tissue regions are described as "dermabrasion." "Microdermabrasion" is designed for local disruption of the SC and superficial viable epidermis (42–45), with minimal to no pain or bleeding and relatively fast recovery time. It is sometimes applied along with topical cosmetic products such as retinoic acid, vitamin C, and nicotinamide (46–48).

Microdermabrasion has also been investigated as a tool for enhancing delivery of therapeutic compounds into the skin. These include locally active ingredients such as 5-fluorouracil, aminolevulinic acid, clobetasol 17-propionate, and systemic drugs such as insulin (44, 49–52). Lee and colleagues utilized a pressurized microdermabrasion system whereby AL_2O_3 microcrystals were propelled onto excised pig skin (49). Lee et al. reported that microdermabrasion by pressurized AL_2O_3 microcrystals significantly improved the flux of 5-fluorouracil across excised pig skin from 1.19 ± 0.82 to 13.16 ± 4.23 $\mu g/cm^2/h$ (an 11.06-fold increase) (49). Microdermabrasion also increased aminolevulinic acid flux by 39-fold in excised pig skin and 48-fold in nude mouse skin. The difference is associated with the thinner and less robust skin of the mouse. In contrast, clobetasol 17-propionate permeation decreased following microdermabrasion. Flux across intact skin was 6.99 ± 3.57, as against 0.56 ± 0.15, 0.94 ± 0.30, and 1.64 ± 0.18 $\mu g/cm^2/h$ following microdermabrasion of 3, 5, and 10 seconds' duration, corresponding to a decrease of approximately 4- to 12-fold. This suggests that while microdermabrasion was an effective skin penetration enhancer for the hydrophilic compounds aminolevulinic acid and fluorouracil (log partition coefficients of 1.5 and −0.89, respectively), it reduced penetration of the lipophilic compound clobetasol 17-propionate (logP of 3.50). This suggests that while removal of the lipid-rich SC benefits penetration of hydrophilic compounds, it reduces penetration of lipophilic compounds. Drugs delivered post-dermabrasion rely on passive diffusion within the viable skin tissue, potentially excluding lipophilic compounds that partition into the now-removed SC lipid bilayers. Controlled microdermabrasion (44, 53) and appropriate vehicle selection tailored to the physicochemistry of the applied compound may allow the technique to be optimized.

5.3.1.1 Thermal Ablation Technologies

Thermal ablation involves heating the skin surface to vaporize SC tissue. If the heating source is effectively controlled, the temperature gradient across the SC can allow extreme heat at the skin surface ($\approx 300°C$ for microseconds) while there is no significant temperature rise in the underlying viable epidermis and deeper skin tissues (54, 55). In effect, this removes portions of the SC to create micron-scale channels similar to those created by a microneedle array. This can be achieved by the application of arrays of microfabricated-resistive (56) and radiofrequency (57, 58) electrical heating elements, and by lasers (following section). The ViaDor™ system (developed by TransPharma Medical, Israel), which creates 144 microchannels in 1 cm^2, is applied followed by patch application. Histological studies demonstrate that the microchannels reach in to the dermis and are almost completely healed within 24 h. A similar technology is the PassPort system (developed by Altea, now owned by Nitto-Denko, Japan and recently spun out as PassPort Technologies Inc, San Diego, CA).

5.3.1.2 Laser Ablation

Laser skin rejuvenation uses devices such as the P.L.E.A.S.E (Painless Laser Epidermal System) for dermatological (scarring, stretch marks) and cosmetic outcomes that apply laser-generated ablative photothermal energy to disrupt and remove the superficial skin layers. These devices cause thermal ablation of the skin using a laser source.

The absorption of laser energy is related to the optical absorbance of water within the skin; thus the choice of laser can be tailored to the depth of desired tissue ablation. A ruby laser has poor water absorbance at 694 nm resulting in a minimally ablative technique, while a CO_2 laser is highly absorbed at 10,600 nm resulting in strong ablation but also more extensive photothermal tissue damage. Erbium:yttrium-gallium-garnet (Er:YAG) and yttrium scandium gallium garnet (YSGG) lasers, emitting at 2790 nm and 2940 nm respectively, offer effective ablation of the SC with reduced thermal damage to the underlying viable tissue (60).

Rather than affect the entire skin surface, fractional laser ablation (59, 61) ablates sub-millimeter regions (spots) within a treatment area interspaced with undamaged tissue, mimicking a microneedle array-type pattern. Average spot size ranges of 40–300 μm with densities between 50 cm^{-2} and 600 cm^{-2} (59, 61–63) correspond to approximately 5% to 30% of disrupted epidermis evenly spaced within a treatment area. The overall effect is minimal photothermal damage and faster healing times due to migration of neighboring viable keratinocytes into the ablated cavities.

Laser ablation has been investigated for delivery of a range of compounds such as imiquimod, 5-aminolevulinic acid, minoxidil, hydro-quinone, nanoparticles, and antigens (59, 61, 62, 64–69). As with all techniques that act by creating pores in the SC, an important consideration is how the properties of the drug and vehicle applied within those pores influence passive diffusion within the skin. Lee et al. (66) reported that penetration enhancement of the relatively lipophilic imiquimod (logP 2.7) of 18.45-fold was achieved when formulated in 40% PEG400 in conjunction with 5 J/cm^2 fluence full skin ablation (ER:YAG). The same formulation applied with a fractional ablation technique (4 J/cm^2 fluence) resulted in a 8.83-fold enhancement. Greater enhancement was achieved with the hydrophilic aminolevulinic acid (logP –1.5). In this case full ablation (2.5 J/cm^2 fluence) resulted in a 641.27-fold and 103.67-fold penetration enhancement when applied in aqueous buffer and 40% PEG respectively. Again, the fractional technique resulted in lower enhancements of 41.23-fold and 0.69-fold in pH 5 buffer and 40% PEG respectively. Clearly, the removal of the SC lipophilic barrier resulted in greater delivery for the hydrophilic than the lipophilic compound. Fractional laser ablation has also been shown to allow effective delivery of 10 kDA dextran, siRNA, and plasmid DNA using both in vitro/in vivo techniques (70) and vaccines (62, 71). While laser ablation can achieve greater delivery rates, it is likely that the lower tissue damage profile of fractional ablation makes this technique more feasible for further development as a skin penetration enhancement technology. However, there would need to be significant technological developments, as current bulky and expensive laser devices are a significant limitation for their further development in the transdermal delivery field.

5.3.2 Biolistic Injectors

5.3.2.1 Liquid Jet Injectors

Jet injectors deliver a liquid payload at high velocity through the skin (Figure 5.5 left). Initial multiuse devices were withdrawn from the market after an outbreak of Hepatitis B due to splashback of bodily fluids onto the surface of the injector (72) and have been replaced by fully disposable single-use injectors (73).

Jet injectors subject the active pharmaceutical ingredient (API) solution to high pressure so that it is ejected through a small nozzle, at velocity greater than 100 m/s, with a maximum of approximately 200 m/s (73). The velocity and microjet size influence the delivered volume and penetration depth of the payload, and also the amount of damage to the skin (73). Deeper penetration is achieved

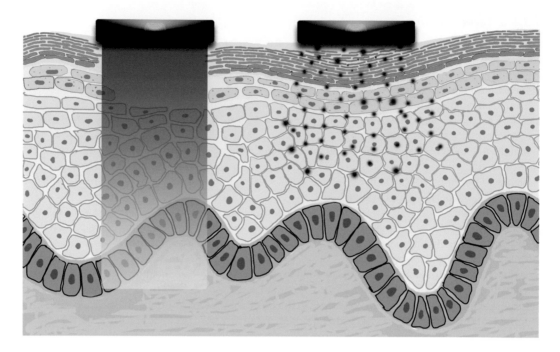

FIGURE 5.5 Biolistic needle-free delivery: (left) liquid jet injector propels active compound solution through the skin layers resulting in broad distribution of the drug; (right) particle delivery (e.g., gene gun) propels nano- or microparticles into the skin at high velocity resulting in deposition within the upper layers.

with higher velocities, but there is also greater potential for splashback of solution from the skin surface.

Stachowiak and colleagues developed a piezoelectric applicator integrated with a conventional glass/stainless steel syringe, allowing an initial high-speed penetration (148 m/s) followed by low-speed delivery (60 m/s) (74). They hypothesized that there would be a linear correlation between the duration of the initial high velocity and penetration depth, thus permitting delivery control and eliminating the problem of splashback. Dynamic delivery of mannitol was analyzed in ex vivo human skin using a high velocity of approximately 200 m/s with the duration increased incrementally from 0 to 5.5 ms. The total combined injection time for the two velocities was 5.5 ms throughout. Optimal mannitol delivery occurred when the high-velocity component was 2–4 ms.

While volumes of up to 250 μL have been delivered (75), these result in more damage to surrounding and deeper skin tissues. Volumes in the nanoliter range minimize damage and splashback (76). Jang and colleagues used an ER:YAG laser to induce a microjet for controlled delivery of epidermal growth factor and human growth hormone (77, 78). A 250-μs laser pulse generated vapour bubbles and downstream shockwaves that propelled the API solution through a nozzle forming a microjet that penetrated the skin. The device was designed with two compartments to prevent any detrimental thermal effects to the API, and to separate the laser-ablation process from the skin. The microjet velocities between 23.0 ± 4.0 and 50.6 ± 1.6 m/s delivered a maximum of 2100 ± 28 nL and minimum of 358 ± 14 nL (an approximately 5.8-fold increase). Delivery of epidermal growth factor and human growth hormone in porcine skin was achieved, as determined by gene expression of keratinocyte laminin and fibroblast elastin respectively. There was no significant difference in gene expression for laser energies of 408 and 816 mJ and two different drug concentrations of 10 and 100 ng/mL suggesting the laser energy caused minimal thermal damage to the API. Continued development of liquid jet injector systems may continue to offer improvements in delivery control with minimal tissue damage, but will need to be achieved at low cost and complexity.

5.3.2.2 Powder/Particulate Injectors

The original biolistic particle delivery system, or gene gun, was designed for delivering exogenous DNA (transgenes) into plant cells. The payload is typically a particle of a heavy metal coated with DNA (typically plasmid DNA). This has been developed into biolistic injectors delivering a "shotgun" burst of nano- or microparticles into the skin (Figure 5.5 right), injectors that have been effective for the immunization of antigens including influenza and malaria, and also in anticancer applications in a range of animals (mice, rat, ferrets, monkeys, etc.) and humans (79–82). Clinical assessment of biolistic particle delivery reports transient localized pain and tissue damage (erythema, irritation, etc.); thus, like liquid biolistic injection, the technique is most suitable to vaccination.

Traditionally, solid or dense particles, preferably spheroidal in the sub-micron-size range were used for biolistic particle delivery (83, 84). However, porous particles can provide an additional option for increased drug loading and controlled release (79).

While both biolistic approaches can deliver their payload into the skin, their sophisticated instrumentation and associated tissue damage is a significant limitation in successful widespread adoption as a transdermal delivery technology. If they have a future it is most likely in the vaccine area.

5.3.2.3 Elongated Microparticles

High-aspect-ratio EMPs (85, 86), for enhanced drug delivery, are made of cylinder-shaped solid silica with an average width of 28 ± 11 μm and an average length between 120.1 and 483.2 μm (Figure 5.6).

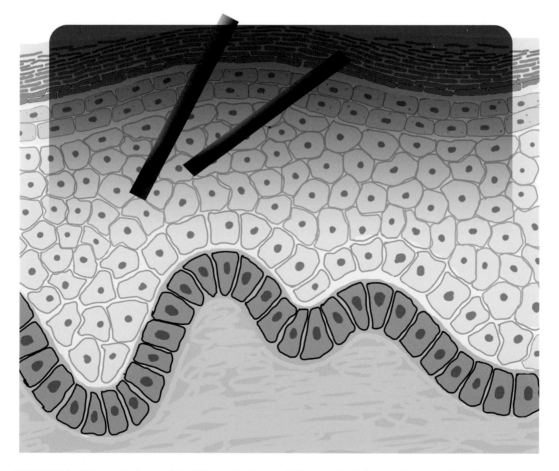

FIGURE 5.6 Elongated microparticle delivery showing the shallow angle of microparticle penetration. The drug can be coated onto or mixed with the microparticles and massaged onto the skin.

EMPs can be mixed with existing formulations and massaged onto the skin; in this case, the EMPs facilitate permeation of the simultaneously applied active in the formulation. Alternative drugs can be coated onto the surface of the EMPs. A 3D-printed micro-textured applicator is used to apply the formulation, maximizing contact with the skin surface at the activation site. Thus, unlike microneedle and other array-type enhancement technologies, EMPs can be applied to varied application site sizes and shapes. Disruption within the epidermis is maximized because the EMPs are designed for low angular penetration within the epidermis, and penetrate to the dermal–epidermal junction (86). The normal transepidermal turnover and desquamation process pushes the microparticles out of healthy skin within 3 weeks.

We have demonstrated a sevenfold increase in delivery of fluorescein to the upper layers of porcine skin using our microparticles when compared to topical application alone and enhanced delivery of therapeutically relevant compounds (vitamins A and B3) in vitro and in vivo (87). In excised human skin, EMPs enhanced vitamin E (3H-a-tocopherol acetate) and vitamin B3 (3H-nicotinamide) delivery by 8.5- and 8.8-fold respectively, compared to topical alone ($p = 0.0017$ and 0.0001) (86). Using confocal microscopy imaging we showed that an average of 76 ± 40 EMPs per mm^2 penetrate the forearm skin of healthy volunteers to an average depth of 48.6 ± 18.4 μm, a formulation of 5 mg of microparticles with 50 μL of 1 mg/mL sodium fluorescein (86). EMPs resulted in a significant 3.3-fold fluorescein delivery increase compared to fluorescein alone, and provided a relatively uniform and continuous delivery profile within the treatment area (86). The EMPs were eliminated from the skin within 3 weeks.

5.4 Comparison of Microneedles with Direct Enhancement Techniques

Direct comparison of the skin delivery efficiency of microneedles and other direct enhancement techniques is difficult, as few comparative studies have been published. While the various techniques have been investigated for a range of small and macromolecules, the experimental protocols vary considerably with differing donor formulations, skin membranes, receptor solutions, etc. Consequently, it is difficult to compare data across the published literature. We conducted a preliminary study to compare the skin penetration of sodium fluorescein applied to excised stillborn piglet skin mounted in Franz-type diffusion cells with microneedles (351 plastic microneedle projections of 650 μm in length; 3M St. Paul, MN), Dermaroller (192 × 0.5 mm stainless steel microneedles in eight rows on the rotating drum; ClinicCare, NSW) and EMP (high-aspect-ratio silica cylinders (diameter 9.3 ± 0.9 μm, length 303.4 ± 208.7 μm). Thus the technologies provided enhancement ratios compared to passive administration of 30, 26 and 19 respectively. All technologies significantly enhanced sodium fluorescein skin penetration compared to passive application (P DermaRoller (20.95 ± 2.53 μg/cm^2) > EMP (15.99 ± 0.97 μg/cm^2) > passive (0.38 ± 0.37 μg/cm^2: Mean $\pm$ SD: $n = 3$). Microneedles provided the greatest enhancement in skin penetration but also exhibited greater variability than the Dermaroller and EMP. Comparison of the amount of sodium fluorescein retained in the skin at 24 h showed a rank order of EMP (9.00 ± 2.09 μg) > DermaRoller (7.17 ± 2.45 μg) > microneedles (3.97 ± 1.71 μg) > passive (2.18 ± 0.97 μg) representing enhancement ratios compared to passive administration of 4.1, 3.3, and 1.8 respectively. In this case, the variability in sodium fluorescein delivery to the skin across the three technologies was similar despite the significantly greater enhancement provided by the EMPs and DermaRoller. This suggests that the choice of technologies may vary depending on the target site for therapeutic outcome.

5.5 Conclusion

Many different strategies have been explored to overcome the SC barrier and increase the therapeutic potential of topical and transdermal delivery. The enhancement technologies described in this chapter have played their part in the greater utilization of the skin as a site of drug application. Microneedles, in their various fabrications, act to create pores through the SC to provide direct access to the viable epidermis and are particularly effective for enhanced delivery of hydrophilic compounds. Other direct methods described in this chapter apply different technologies but essentially also work on the principle of creating pores through the SC. The direct enhancement technologies have particular promise in the delivery of macromolecules such as vaccines, but also have potential to increase the dosages of all drugs that can be administered and may also have particular utility for targeting drugs to skin lesions (87). Some of the indirect physical methods discussed also provide significant SC barrier reduction though they do not create pores comparable to microneedling. The combination of microneedling with other technologies may offer more delivery but can be associated with definite costs such as increased complexity/cost and confounding results. The goal of such a combination is always potentiation, but the reality may just be additive. The aim of this chapter is to discuss the alternative enhancement technologies to microneedles. The potential to combine technologies with microneedles is explored in a subsequent chapter. Microneedling and comparable technologies offer great promise for future development. We will likely see continued technological advances to permit scale-up and manufacturing in an efficient and cost-effective manner, and the combination of enhancement strategies to maximize delivery.

REFERENCES

1. Yu J, Zhang Y, Ye Y, DiSanto R, Sun W, Ranson D, Ligler FS, Buse JB, Gu Z. Microneedle-array patches loaded with hypoxia-sensitive vesicles provide fast glucose-responsive insulin delivery. Proceedings of the national academy of sciences of the United States of America. 2015;112(27):8260–8265.
2. Lee H, Song C, Hong YS, Kim MS, Cho HR, Kang T, Shin K, Choi SH, Hyeon T, Kim DH. Wearable/disposable sweat-based glucose monitoring device with multistage transdermal drug delivery module. Science advances. 2017;3(3):e1601314.
3. Kalia YN, Naik A, Garrison J, Guy RH. Iontophoretic drug delivery. Advanced drug delivery reviews. 2004;56(5):619–658.
4. Marro D, Kalia YN, Delgado-Charro MB, Guy RH. Contributions of electromigration and electroosmosis to iontophoretic drug delivery. Pharmaceutical research. 2001;18(12):1701–1708.
5. Guy RH, Kalia YN, Delgado-Charro MB, Merino V, Lopez A, Marro D. Iontophoresis: electrorepulsion and electroosmosis. Journal of controlled release. 2000;64(1–3):129–132.
6. Gratieri T, Kalaria D, Kalia YN. Non-invasive iontophoretic delivery of peptides and proteins across the skin. Expert opinion on drug delivery. 2011;8(5):645–663.
7. Sieg A, Wascotte V. Diagnostic and therapeutic applications of iontophoresis. Journal of drug targeting. 2009;17(9):690–700.
8. Roustit M, Blaise S, Cracowski JL. Trials and tribulations of skin iontophoresis in therapeutics. British journal of clinical pharmacology. 2014;77(1):63–71.
9. Denet AR, Vanbever R, Preat V. Skin electroporation for transdermal and topical delivery. Advanced drug delivery reviews. 2004;56(5):659–674.
10. Hooper JW, Golden JW, Ferro AM, King AD. Smallpox DNA vaccine delivered by novel skin electroporation device protects mice against intranasal poxvirus challenge. Vaccine. 2007;25(10):1814–1823.
11. Rosati M, Valentin A, Jalah R, Patel V, von Gegerfelt A, Bergamaschi C, Alicea C, Weiss D, Treece J, Pal R, Markham PD, Marques ET, August JT, Khan A, Draghia-Akli R, Felber BK, Pavlakis GN. Increased immune responses in rhesus macaques by DNA vaccination combined with electroporation. Vaccine. 2008;26(40):5223–5229.
12. Bodles-Brakhop AM, Heller R, Draghia-Akli R. Electroporation for the delivery of DNA-based vaccines and immunotherapeutics: current clinical developments. Molecular therapy. 2009;17(4):585–592.
13. Gothelf A, Gehl J. Electroporation-based DNA delivery technology: methods for gene electrotransfer to skin. Methods in molecular biology. 2014;1143:115–122.
14. Shen X, Soderholm J, Lin F, Kobinger G, Bello A, Gregg DA, Broderick KE, Sardesai NY. Influenza A vaccines using linear expression cassettes delivered via electroporation afford full protection against challenge in a mouse model. Vaccine. 2012;30(48):6946–6954.
15. Johansson DX, Ljungberg K, Kakoulidou M, Liljestrom P. Intradermal electroporation of naked replicon RNA elicits strong immune responses. PloS one. 2012;7(1):e29732.
16. Zorec B, Becker S, Rebersek M, Miklavcic D, Pavselj N. Skin electroporation for transdermal drug delivery: the influence of the order of different square wave electric pulses. International journal of pharmaceutics. 2013;457(1):214–223.

17. Murthy SN, Sammeta SM, Bowers C. Magnetophoresis for enhancing transdermal drug delivery: mechanistic studies and patch design. Journal of controlled release. 2010;148(2):197–203.

18. Namjoshi S, Cacetta R, Edwards J, Benson HA. Liquid chromatography assay for 5-aminolevulinic acid: application to in vitro assessment of skin penetration via Dermaportation. Journal of chromatography B, Analytical technologies in the biomedical and life sciences. 2007;852(1–2):49–55.

19. Krishnan G, Edwards J, Chen Y, Benson HAE. Enhanced skin permeation of naltrexone by pulsed electromagnetic fields in human skin in vitro. Journal of pharmaceutical sciences. 2010;99(6):2724–2731.

20. Namjoshi S, Chen Y, Edwards J, Benson HA. Enhanced transdermal delivery of a dipeptide by dermaportation. Biopolymers. 2008;90(5):655–662.

21. Mohammed YH, Yamada M, Lin LL, Grice JE, Roberts MS, Raphael AP, Benson HA, Prow TW. Microneedle enhanced delivery of cosmeceutically relevant peptides in human skin. PloS one. 2014;9(7):e101956.

22. Polat BE, Hart D, Langer R, Blankschtein D. Ultrasound-mediated transdermal drug delivery: mechanisms, scope, and emerging trends. Journal of controlled release. 2011;152(3):330–348.

23. Azagury A, Khoury L, Enden G, Kost J. Ultrasound mediated transdermal drug delivery. Advanced drug delivery reviews. 2014;72:127–143.

24. Krasovitski B, Frenkel V, Shoham S, Kimmel E. Intramembrane cavitation as a unifying mechanism for ultrasound-induced bioeffects. Proceedings of the national academy of sciences of the United States of America. 2011;108(8):3258–3263.

25. Mitragotri S, Blankschtein D, Langer R. Ultrasound-mediated transdermal protein delivery. Science. 1995;269(5225):850–853.

26. Tezel A, Paliwal S, Shen Z, Mitragotri S. Low-frequency ultrasound as a transcutaneous immunization adjuvant. Vaccine. 2005;23(29):3800–3807.

27. Dahlan A, Alpar HO, Stickings P, Sesardic D, Murdan S. Transcutaneous immunisation assisted by low-frequency ultrasound. International journal of pharmaceutics. 2009;368(1–2):123–128.

28. Smith NB, Lee S, Shung KK. Ultrasound-mediated transdermal in vivo transport of insulin with low-profile cymbal arrays. Ultrasound in medicine & biology. 2003;29(8):1205–1210.

29. Luis J, Park EJ, Meyer RJ, Smith NB. Rectangular cymbal arrays for improved ultrasonic transdermal insulin delivery. Journal of the acoustical society of America. 2007;122(4):2022–2030.

30. Park EJ, Werner J, Beebe J, Chan S, Smith NB. Noninvasive ultrasonic glucose sensing with large pigs (approximately 200 pounds) using a lightweight cymbal transducer array and biosensors. Journal of diabetes science and technology. 2009;3(3):517–523.

31. Schoellhammer CM, Polat BE, Mendenhall J, Maa R, Jones B, Hart DP, Langer R, Blankschtein D. Rapid skin permeabilization by the simultaneous application of dual-frequency, high-intensity ultrasound. Journal of controlled release. 2012;163(2):154–160.

32. Saletes I, Gilles B, Bera JC. Promoting inertial cavitation by nonlinear frequency mixing in a bifrequency focused ultrasound beam. Ultrasonics. 2011;51(1):94–101.

33. Lee S, McAuliffe DJ, Flotte TJ, Kollias N, Doukas AG. Photomechanical transdermal delivery: the effect of laser confinement. Lasers in surgery and medicine. 2001;28(4):344–347.

34. Lee WR, Shen SC, Wang KH, Hu CH, Fang JY. The effect of laser treatment on skin to enhance and control transdermal delivery of 5-fluorouracil. Journal of pharmaceutical sciences. 2002;91(7):1613–1626.

35. Lee S, McAuliffe DJ, Kollias N, Flotte TJ, Doukas AG. Photomechanical delivery of 100-nm microspheres through the stratum corneum: implications for transdermal drug delivery. Lasers in surgery and medicine. 2002;31(3):207–210.

36. Doukas AG, Kollias N. Transdermal drug delivery with a pressure wave. Advanced drug delivery reviews. 2004;56(5):559–579.

37. Lee S, McAuliffe DJ, Flotte TJ, Kollias N, Doukas AG. Photomechanical transcutaneous delivery of macromolecules. Journal of investigative dermatology. 1998;111(6):925–929.

38. Lee S, McAuliffe DJ, Kollias N, Flotte TJ, Doukas AG. Permeabilization and recovery of the stratum corneum in vivo: the synergy of photomechanical waves and sodium lauryl sulfate. Lasers in surgery and medicine. 2001;29(2):145–150.

39. Lee S, McAuliffe DJ, Mulholland SE, Doukas AG. Photomechanical transdermal delivery of insulin in vivo. Lasers in surgery and medicine. 2001;28(3):282–285.
40. Nguyen T. Dermatology procedures: microdermabrasion and chemical peels. FP essentials. 2014;426:16–23.
41. Karimipour DJ, Karimipour G, Orringer JS. Microdermabrasion: an evidence-based review. Plastic and reconstructive surgery. 2010;125(1):372–377.
42. Freedman BM, Rueda-Pedraza E, Earley RV. Clinical and histologic changes determine optimal treatment regimens for microdermabrasion. Journal of dermatological treatment. 2002;13(4):193–200.
43. Andrews S, Lee JW, Prausnitz M. Recovery of skin barrier after stratum corneum removal by microdermabrasion. AAPS pharmSciTech. 2011;12(4):1393–1400.
44. Andrews S, Lee JW, Choi SO, Prausnitz MR. Transdermal insulin delivery using microdermabrasion. Pharmaceutical research. 2011;28(9):2110–2118.
45. Andrews SN, Zarnitsyn V, Bondy B, Prausnitz MR. Optimization of microdermabrasion for controlled removal of stratum corneum. International journal of pharmaceutics. 2011;407(1-2):95–104.
46. Hexsel D, Mazzuco R, Dal'Forno T, Zechmeister D. Microdermabrasion followed by a 5% retinoid acid chemical peel vs. a 5% retinoid acid chemical peel for the treatment of photoaging—a pilot study. Journal of cosmetic dermatology. 2005;4(2):111–116.
47. Zhou Y, Banga AK. Enhanced delivery of cosmeceuticals by microdermabrasion. Journal of cosmetic dermatology. 2011;10(3):179–184.
48. Lee WR, Shen SC, Kuo-Hsien W, Hu CH, Fang JY. Lasers and microdermabrasion enhance and control topical delivery of vitamin C. The journal of investigative dermatology. 2003;121(5):1118–1125.
49. Lee WR, Tsai RY, Fang CL, Liu CJ, Hu CH, Fang JY. Microdermabrasion as a novel tool to enhance drug delivery via the skin: an animal study. Dermatologic surgery. 2006;32(8):1013–1022.
50. Linkner RV, Jim On S, Haddican M, Singer G, Shim-Chang H. Evaluating the efficacy of photodynamic therapy with 20% aminolevulinic acid and microdermabrasion as a combination treatment regimen for acne scarring: a split-face, randomized, double-blind pilot study. Journal of clinical and aesthetic dermatology. 2014;7(5):32–35.
51. Garg T, Chander R, Jain A. Combination of microdermabrasion and 5-fluorouracil to induce repigmentation in vitiligo: an observational study. Dermatologic surgery. 2011;37(12):1763–1766.
52. Andrews SN, Jeong E, Prausnitz MR. Transdermal delivery of molecules is limited by full epidermis, not just stratum corneum. Pharmaceutical research. 2013;30(4):1099–1109.
53. Gill HS, Andrews SN, Sakthivel SK, Fedanov A, Williams IR, Garber DA, Priddy FH, Yellin S, Feinberg MB, Staprans SI, Prausnitz MR. Selective removal of stratum corneum by microdermabrasion to increase skin permeability. European journal of pharmaceutical sciences. 2009;38(2):95–103.
54. Park JH, Lee JW, Kim YC, Prausnitz MR. The effect of heat on skin permeability. International journal of pharmaceutics. 2008;359(1–2):94–103.
55. Lee JW, Gadiraju P, Park JH, Allen MG, Prausnitz MR. Microsecond thermal ablation of skin for transdermal drug delivery. Journal of controlled release. 2011;154(1):58–68.
56. Bramson J, Dayball K, Evelegh C, Wan YH, Page D, Smith A. Enabling topical immunization via microporation: a novel method for pain-free and needle-free delivery of adenovirus-based vaccines. Gene therapy. 2003;10(3):251–260.
57. Sintov AC, Krymberk I, Daniel D, Hannan T, Sohn Z, Levin G. Radiofrequency-driven skin microchanneling as a new way for electrically assisted transdermal delivery of hydrophilic drugs. Journal of controlled release. 2003;89(2):311–320.
58. Levin G, Gershonowitz A, Sacks H, Stern M, Sherman A, Rudaev S, Zivin I, Phillip M. Transdermal delivery of human growth hormone through RF-microchannels. Pharmaceutical research. 2005;22(4):550–555.
59. Haak CS, Farinelli WA, Tam J, Doukas AG, Anderson RR, Haedersdal M. Fractional laser-assisted delivery of methyl aminolevulinate: impact of laser channel depth and incubation time. Lasers in surgery and medicine. 2012;44(10):787–795.
60. Lin CH, Aljuffali IA, Fang JY. Lasers as an approach for promoting drug delivery via skin. Expert opinion on drug delivery. 2014;11(4):599–614.

61. Rkein A, Ozog D, Waibel JS. Treatment of atrophic scars with fractionated CO_2 laser facilitating delivery of topically applied poly-L-lactic acid. Dermatologic surgery. 2014;40(6):624–631.
62. Scheiblhofer S, Thalhamer J, Weiss R. Laser microporation of the skin: prospects for painless application of protective and therapeutic vaccines. Expert opinion on drug delivery. 2013;10(6):761–773.
63. Helsing P, Togsverd-Bo K, Veierod MB, Mork G, Haedersdal M. Intensified fractional CO_2 laser-assisted photodynamic therapy vs. laser alone for organ transplant recipients with multiple actinic keratoses and wart-like lesions: a randomized half-side comparative trial on dorsal hands. British journal of dermatology. 2013;169(5):1087–1092.
64. Yu J, Kalaria DR, Kalia YN. Erbium:YAG fractional laser ablation for the percutaneous delivery of intact functional therapeutic antibodies. Journal of controlled release. 2011;156(1):53–59.
65. Lee WR, Shen SC, Aljuffali IA, Li YC, Fang JY. Impact of different vehicles for laser-assisted drug permeation via skin: full-surface versus fractional ablation. Pharmaceutical research. 2014;31(2): 382–393.
66. Lee WR, Shen SC, Aljuffali IA, Li YC, Fang JY. Erbium-yttrium-aluminum-garnet laser irradiation ameliorates skin permeation and follicular delivery of antialopecia drugs. Journal of pharmaceutical sciences. 2014;103(11):3542–3552.
67. Kauvar AN. Successful treatment of melasma using a combination of microdermabrasion and Q-switched Nd:YAG lasers. Lasers in surgery and medicine. 2012;44(2):117–124.
68. Kauvar AN. The evolution of melasma therapy: targeting melanosomes using low-fluence Q-switched neodymium-doped yttrium aluminium garnet lasers. Seminars in cutaneous medicine and surgery. 2012;31(2):126–132.
69. Haedersdal M, Sakamoto FH, Farinelli WA, Doukas AG, Tam J, Anderson RR. Pretreatment with ablative fractional laser changes kinetics and biodistribution of topical 5-aminolevulinic acid (ALA) and methyl aminolevulinate (MAL). Lasers in surgery and medicine. 2014;46(6):462–469.
70. Lee WR, Shen SC, Chen WY, Aljuffali IA, Suen SY, Fang JY. Noninvasive delivery of siRNA and plasmid DNA into skin by fractional ablation: erbium:YAG laser versus CO(2) laser. European journal of pharmaceutics and biopharmaceutics. 2014;86(3):315–323.
71. Scheiblhofer S, Strobl A, Hoepflinger V, Thalhamer T, Steiner M, Thalhamer J, Weiss R. Skin vaccination via fractional infrared laser ablation—optimization of laser-parameters and adjuvantation. Vaccine. 2017;35(14):1802–1809.
72. Giudice EL, Campbell JD. Needle-free vaccine delivery. Advanced drug delivery reviews. 2006;58(1):68–89.
73. Mitragotri S. Current status and future prospects of needle-free liquid jet injectors. Nature reviews. Drug discovery. 2006;5(7):543–548.
74. Stachowiak JC, Li TH, Arora A, Mitragotri S, Fletcher DA. Dynamic control of needle-free jet injection. Journal of controlled release. 2009;135(2):104–112.
75. Taberner A, Hogan NC, Hunter IW. Needle-free jet injection using real-time controlled linear Lorentz-force actuators. Medical engineering & physics. 2012;34(9):1228–1235.
76. Park MA, Jang HJ, Sirotkin FV, Yoh JJ. Er:YAG laser pulse for small-dose splashback-free microjet transdermal drug delivery. Optics letters. 2012;37(18):3894–3896.
77. Jang HJ, Hur E, Kim Y, Lee SH, Kang NG, Yoh JJ. Laser-induced microjet injection into preablated skin for more effective transdermal drug delivery. Journal of biomedical optics. 2014;19(11):118002.
78. Jang HJ, Yu H, Lee S, Hur E, Kim Y, Lee SH, Kang N, Yoh JJ. Towards clinical use of a laser-induced microjet system aimed at reliable and safe drug delivery. Journal of biomedical optics. 2014;19(5):058001.
79. Zilony N, Tzur-Balter A, Segal E, Shefi O. Bombarding cancer: biolistic delivery of therapeutics using porous Si carriers. Scientific reports. 2013;3:2499.
80. Bergmann-Leitner ES, Leitner WW. Improving DNA vaccines against malaria: could immunization by gene gun be the answer? Therapeutic delivery. 2013;4(7):767–770.
81. Wang S, Zhang C, Zhang L, Li J, Huang Z, Lu S. The relative immunogenicity of DNA vaccines delivered by the intramuscular needle injection, electroporation and gene gun methods. Vaccine. 2008;26(17):2100–2110.
82. Bragstad K, Martel CJ, Thomsen JS, Jensen KL, Nielsen LP, Aasted B, Fomsgaard A. Pandemic influenza 1918 H1N1 and 1968 H3N2 DNA vaccines induce cross-reactive immunity in ferrets against infection with viruses drifted for decades. Influenza and other respiratory viruses. 2011;5(1):13–23.

83. Kendall M, Mitchell T, Wrighton-Smith P. Intradermal ballistic delivery of micro-particles into excised human skin for pharmaceutical applications. Journal of biomechanics. 2004;37(11): 1733–1741.

84. Liu Y, Kendall MA. Optimization of a jet-propelled particle injection system for the uniform transdermal delivery of drug/vaccine. Biotechnology and bioengineering. 2007;97(5):1300–1308.

85. Raphael AP, Primiero CA, Lin LL, Smith RF, Dyer P, Soyer HP, Prow TW. High aspect ratio elongated microparticles for enhanced topical drug delivery in human volunteers. Advanced healthcare materials. 2014.

86. Raphael AP, Primiero CA, Ansaldo AB, Keates HL, Soyer HP, Prow TW. Elongate microparticles for enhanced drug delivery to ex vivo and in vivo pig skin. Journal of controlled release. 2013;172(1):96–104.

87. Yamada M, Prow TW. Physical drug delivery enhancement for aged skin, UV damaged skin and skin cancer: Translation and commercialization. Adv Drug Deliv Rev. 2020 Apr(24:S0169–409X(20)30028-4. doi: 10.1016/j.addr.2020.04.008.

6

Combination of Microneedles with Other Methods

Sahitya Katikaneni
Zosano Pharma

6.1 Introduction

The most common route of drug delivery to date is oral; the second most common is parenteral adminis-tration. Drug delivery through skin provides an excellent opportunity to overcome issues with other routes of administration such as hepatic and gastric degradation, needle phobia, and pain (1). The past decade has seen major advancements in the field of microneedle-mediated transdermal delivery, all thanks to the research conducted by academic groups and pharmaceutical companies worldwide. Microneedles have proven more effective compared to other technologies as far as skin delivery is concerned (1). The ability of microneedles to temporarily create micron-sized pores in the skin has even made it possible to deliver hydrophilic and high-molecular-weight compounds such as proteins and vaccines through skin (2–5). Other transdermal technologies such as iontophoresis and ultrasound have been shown to deliver such molecules as well, but have size limitations (1, 6, 7). Microporation has also found relevance in diagnostic testing, as it can enable sampling of biological fluids for monitoring blood glucose levels (5). Application of advanced engineering tools in the fabrication of microneedles has opened up endless opportunities to design the type of delivery for the desired therapeutic effect (4). Immediate release with coated microneedles (metal/dissolvable), controlled release from microneedles containing encapsulated drug, and infusion through hollow microneedles are a few potential ways of drug administration with microneedles (4).

Microneedles can comprise different materials: metals such as stainless steel and titanium, polymers such as poly(lactic-co-glycolic acid) (PLGA) and carboxy methyl cellulose, or sugars such as maltose and dextrin (2, 3, 5, 8–12). They can be either hollow or solid and can be made in a wide variety of geometries as per the application. They can be applied to the skin manually or with the aid of a special device (4, 13, 14). Combining microneedles with other technologies might exhibit a synergistic response on delivery. Several groups have published their research in this area and are continuing to gather data. This chapter focuses on the combinatorial aspect and looks into combination of microneedle technology with other methods.

6.2 Combination of Microneedles with Other Technologies

6.2.1 Iontophoresis

Transdermal iontophoresis refers to application of physiologically acceptable electric current (< 0.5 mA/cm^2) to enable movement of charged or ionized molecules into or across a membrane (15). This delivery method is suitable for polar molecules with high charge density. The amount of drug delivered via iontophoresis is proportional to the intensity of the current applied across the tissue (15). Iontophoretic transport is governed by two major mechanisms, electromigration and electroosmosis. Detailed information on the transport mechanisms and specific applications of iontophoresis can be found in these review articles (6, 15–17). One of the key features of iontophoretic delivery is its ability to be tailored to an individual's dose requirements. Drugs can be delivered in a continuous or a pulsatile fashion by programming the current (15). However, there are limitations to iontophoresis, one of the biggest of which is that it can only deliver molecules up to approximately 15 kDa in size (18–22).

As mentioned previously, microneedles perturb the skin barrier function in a reversible manner, enabling delivery of macromolecules. The combination of microneedles with iontophoresis will further broaden the scope of molecules that can be delivered via skin. Programmable delivery across pores created by microneedles will help personalize the delivery system to suit one's needs.

In a study conducted by Lin et al., transdermal delivery of an antisense oligonucleotide was evaluated using a combination of microneedles and iontophoresis. Microneedles were made up of stainless steel with a length of 430 μm. The patch size was 2 cm^2 and the current density applied was 100 μA/cm^2. The study was conducted in hairless guinea pig model in vivo. The skin flux was found to be 100 times higher with the combination approach than iontophoresis alone. In spite of oligonucleotides being charged molecules, therapeutic levels were attained only upon combining iontophoretic delivery with microneedles (23).

Wu et al. evaluated in vitro skin permeation of high-molecular-weight fluorescent tagged dextran molecules FD-4, FD-10, FD-40, FD-70, FD-2000 corresponding to an average molecular weight of 3.8, 10.1, 39.0, 71.2, 200 kDa. Studies were performed across hairless rat skin using a combination of microneedles and iontophoresis. Delivery was found to be higher for the combination of microneedles with iontophoresis compared to iontophoresis alone. Permeation was approximately 14-, 26-, 12-, 7- and 14-fold higher for FD-4, FD-10, FD-40, FD-70, and FD-2000 respectively for the combination approach (19).

Transdermal permeation of low-molecular-weight heparin was evaluated by Lanke et al. in an in vitro study. Skin flux with iontophoresis alone was minimal. However, iontophoresis across microneedle-treated skin resulted in flux enhancement by 15-fold. It was mentioned in the study that low-molecular-weight heparin interacts with stratum corneum, and hence methods like microporation in which stratum corneum is disrupted briefly aided in the skin permeation. Combining iontophoresis with microneedles therefore resulted in an additive effect (24).

Delivery of methotrexate (molecular weight 454 Da) was studied in vitro and in vivo by Vemulapalli et al. (21). Delivery was enhanced by 25-fold with the combination of microneedles and iontophoresis as compared to them individually. They also evaluated permeation of salmon calcitonin in vivo. Maltose microneedles were used to pretreat the skin. A current density of 0.2 mA/cm^2 was applied for 1 h. Microneedles alone resulted in a 2.5-fold increase in delivery as compared to iontophoresis. However, the combination of microneedles and iontophoresis resulted in a ninefold enhancement (20).

Katikaneni et al. studied the in vitro delivery of a 13-kDa peptide using the combination with respect to the mechanism dominating the transport during iontophoresis (22). Tape stripping wherein the stratum corneum is completely removed resulted in a complete impairment of electroosmosis, thus altering the skin's permselective properties. This study showed that partial breaching of the skin barrier as it happens during microporation did not impede electroosmosis. In vitro skin flux of the peptide was found to be higher when microneedles and iontophoresis were used in conjunction. A total cumulative amount of 700 ng/cm^2 and 25 μg/cm^2 of the peptide was delivered for the two formulations evaluated at pH 7.5 and pH 4.0 respectively. There were no detectable levels of the peptide when iontophoresis was applied across intact skin. It was established in this case that delivery across microporated skin was higher when electrorepulsion was the dominant force during iontophoresis as compared to electroosmosis. An in vivo study conducted on the same peptide resulted in similar results (25). Daniplestim concentration in the patch was 2 mg/mL. Combination of microneedles and iontophoresis resulted in a C_{max} of about 9 ng/mL. Peptide delivery with iontophoresis or microneedles alone was negligible.

6.2.2 Sonophoresis

Delivery of therapeutic molecules into or across the skin using ultrasound is referred to as sonophoresis or phonophoresis. High-frequency ultrasound (> 0.7 MHz) was used in early investigations and enhancement in permeation anywhere between 1- and 10-fold were seen. However, the past two decades have focused on using low-frequency ultrasound (20–100 kHz) for transdermal delivery along with the development of a better mechanistic understanding of sonophoresis (26, 27). Low-frequency and high-frequency ultrasound differ in the way they facilitate skin permeabilization. The primary mode of enhancement with low-frequency ultrasound is believed to be acoustic cavitation above the skin membrane and for high-frequency ultrasound it is believed to be cavitation within the skin. High-frequency ultrasound has been found to be more effective in increasing the skin permeation of low-molecular-weight compounds whereas low-frequency ultrasound has been more effective in delivering macromolecules such as proteins, vaccines, and nanoparticles. A review article by Polat et al. provides a detailed understanding of the history, mechanistic aspects, and applications of ultrasound for transdermal delivery (7).

There are two ways of applying ultrasound to the skin: (i) a pretreatment approach wherein ultrasound is applied to the skin and followed by application of the drug patch and (ii) a concurrent approach wherein ultrasound is simultaneously applied through the coupling medium containing the drug. Method (i) is more widely followed as simultaneous application of ultrasound may result in drug degradation or cause other undesirable effects. Some of the parameters that influence delivery during ultrasound are the treatment time, duty cycle, distance between the ultrasound transducer and the skin, and the composition of the coupling medium. Combination of ultrasound with microneedles can provide an interesting platform for drug delivery. However, research in this area is in the nascent stage and limited data is available so far.

Hollow microneedles can be applied to the skin and ultrasound can be applied simultaneously so that it can enhance delivery by convection. A study conducted by Chen et al. has used this concept to deliver bovine serum albumin (BSA) and calcein (28). They used hollow microneedles with a length of 100 μm. The frequency of the ultrasound applied was 20 kHz with a cycle length of 10 μs. The ultrasound transducer was attached to the back of the microneedle patch. Skin permeation was enhanced 9 times for calcein and 12 times for BSA as compared to passive diffusion.

Solid or dissolvable microneedles can be used to create pores in the skin. Application of ultrasound on the pretreated skin will result in permeation enhancement due to cavitational effects induced by the ultrasound. This concept was evaluated in a study conducted by Han and Das for delivery of BSA. Solid microneedles with two different lengths, 1.2 mm and 1.5 mm, were used to pretreat the skin. Ultrasound with a frequency of 20 kHz was applied for 10 min.

BSA permeation was more with the combination of microneedles and ultrasound as compared to microneedles or ultrasound alone. Maximum enhancement was achieved when combined with 1.5-mm-long microneedles (29).

Another approach that has been suggested in this area is to pretreat the skin with high-intensity ultrasound followed by application of short-length microneedles. This concept can be used for topical delivery of drugs or for molecules that need a rapid onset of action (30).

6.2.3 Electroporation

Skin electroporation refers to application of high-voltage electric pulses (typically 5–1000 V/cm) for a short duration resulting in formation of aqueous pores in the skin. High electric pulses when applied result in a temporary modification of the stratum corneum resulting in increased electrophoretic mobility and molecular diffusivity. This technique has been shown to improve skin permeability of drug molecules with various lipophilicities and sizes. It is believed to be applicable for both ionic and nonionic molecules. Skin delivery of high molecular weight compounds like peptides, proteins, and oligonucleotides has also been evaluated using electroporation. Detailed mechanistic understanding of skin electroporation and applications with respect to transdermal drug delivery are presented in an excellent review by Kevin Ita (31).

Transdermal delivery of drugs using electroporation has been widely tested in animals, but data in humans is limited (1, 32, 33). Combining electroporation with microneedles may have a beneficial effect on enhancing skin flux. This strategy has not been well tested and needs to be explored further.

Wilke et al. designed a novel drug delivery system called ENDOPORATOR that combined microneedles with electroporation. The device consisted of hollow silicon microneedle electrode arrays with attached sensors. Microneedles penetrate the skin while electroporation will enable injection/infusion of drugs through the needles into the skin (34).

In a study conducted by Hooper et al., delivery of smallpox DNA vaccine was studied using a combination of electroporation and microneedles. Plasmid DNA was coated onto the microneedles and applied to the skin. The dissolved DNA would permeate into the cells with the help of electroporation. The immune response obtained in mice which were vaccinated with this approach was better than the response seen in mice vaccinated with traditional live virus (35).

Delivery of FITC-Dextran with a molecular weight of 4.3 kDa was evaluated in vitro by Yan et al. Skin was pretreated with microneedles followed by application of high-voltage pulses using electrodes. Two types of electroporation were tested: *in-skin* and *on-skin*. Delivery was found to be higher with the combination approach for both the electroporation methods when compared to microneedles or electroporation alone. Delivery was found to be dependent on voltage and pulse width. Permeability with on-skin electroporation was 20-fold higher and with in-skin electroporation it was 140-fold higher. No significant skin irritation was observed (36).

6.2.4 Particulate Systems

Particulate systems (nanoparticles and microparticles) for drug delivery have been thoroughly explored in the past decade. These systems vary in their size and physicochemical properties depending on the material of origin such as lipids, sugars, or polymers (37). They offer several advantages over conventional delivery systems such as: (i) drug release for a prolonged/defined period of time, (ii) enabling of site-specific action by targeting the desired organ/tissue, (iii) providing protection to the drug molecule from proteolytic or mucosal degradation by encapsulating it, thus increasing bioavailability (1, 37–41).

Transdermal delivery of nanoparticles has been mainly used to deliver drugs to the skin for local effects. The mechanism of skin penetration for nanoparticles is not clear; however, hair follicles and furrows are believed to be the potential sites (42). Delivery of nanoparticles into deeper layers of skin without compromising its barrier properties has been challenging. As microporation results in formation of micron-sized pathways in the skin, delivery of nanoparticles beyond the stratum corneum might be possible. However, limited work has been published in this aspect.

6.2.4.1 Solid Microneedles

McAllister et al. published a first report on delivery of latex nanospheres through skin using microneedles (43). Molecules of different radii such as calcein, insulin, BSA, and nanospheres were evaluated in this in vitro study using solid microneedles. Human cadaver epidermis was pretreated with microneedles. Without microporation, there were no detectable levels of any of the above-mentioned molecules. With pretreatment, molecular diffusion on the order of 0.001–0.01 cm/h was seen depending on the molecular radius of the molecule. Highest diffusion was seen for calcein and the lowest for nanospheres. Mechanism of permeation of the nanoparticles was evaluated using mathematical modeling. It supported the theory that diffusion happens through the water-filled channels created in the skin by microneedles.

In a study conducted by Coulman et al., diffusion of latex fluorescent nanospheres (100–150 nm diameter) was evaluated (44). Skin was pretreated with silicon microneedles following application of nanospheres to the skin. Results suggested that the nanospheres migrated into microchannels and to the cells of the epidermis. Similar results were obtained in a study conducted by Chabri et al. (45). Intradermal delivery of polystyrene nanoparticles of approximately 100 nm in diameter was possible through the microchannels. In another study, nanoparticles were found in the epidermis following application of hydrogel/nanoparticle formulation in combination with microneedles (46).

Verbaan et al. evaluated an electrical applicator to apply microneedles with a preset speed. Various speeds were experimented with fluorescein isothiocyanate (FITC)-tagged nanoparticles with a size of 200 nm. Results indicated that nanoparticles were seen in the conduits irrespective of the speeds tested (14).

Delivery of PLGA nanoparticles loaded with coumarin 6 was studied by Zhang et al. Solid silicon microneedles were used for pretreating the skin. Nanoparticles were found significantly in the epidermis compared to dermis and the diffusion rate of nanoparticles was found to be dependent on the concentration of the nanoparticles (47).

Gomaa et al. studied permeation of PLGA nanoparticles across porcine skin pretreated with polymeric microneedles. Permeation of nanoparticles was believed to be dependent on particle size, surface charge, and composition (48).

6.2.4.2 Hollow Microneedles

Wang et al. conducted a study to evaluate the ability to inject particles intradermally using hollow microneedles (49). Two different sizes of microparticles were tested 2.5 um and 2.8 um. They were injected using a single hollow glass microneedle. Particles were successfully injected both ex vivo and in vivo into hairless rat skin. Similarly, in another study hollow silicon microneedles were used to inject an aqueous suspension of blue and fluorescent polystyrene microspheres (50). Observation using confocal microscopy suggested that particles were detected at a depth of 70 um. However, the majority of the particles were found to be 20 um from the surface of the skin.

6.2.4.3 Application in Drug and Vaccine Delivery

Several research groups have studied skin delivery of insulin using a combination of microneedles and nano- or microparticles (51–53). In a study conducted by Ito et al., in mice, insulin was formulated into chondroitin sulfate matrix and adsorbed onto two different types of porous microparticles (51). A control comprising microneedles containing free insulin was included in the study. Blood samples were collected from mice 8 h post-application for all treatment groups. A greater hypoglycemic effect was seen with insulin–microparticle group compared to free insulin group. A "smart insulin patch" was developed by Yu et al. It basically consisted of a microneedle array containing glucose-responsive vesicles loaded with insulin in the tip (53). A chemical reaction at the local site would trigger dissociation of vesicles leading to release of insulin. In vivo testing of this patch in a Type I diabetes mouse model indicated that these arrays were able to control glucose levels over a period of few hours.

Skin is a very effective site for vaccination due to the presence of dendritic cells and Langerhans cells in the epidermal region. Use of particle-based vaccine formulations could be advantageous owing to their inherent immunogenic properties as showcased by several research groups (54). They also have the ability to stabilize the antigen and protect it from any degradation (55–58). Also, they can provide controlled release depending on the need. However, there might be exceptions, and several factors such as physical, chemical properties of the antigen or particle matrix might influence the final result. A study conducted by Bal et al. evaluated the delivery and immunogenicity of diphtheria toxoid with N-trimethyl chitosan as the adjuvant. The vaccine nanoparticles were coated onto solid metallic microneedles. Upon application, nanoparticles would deposit in the skin and act as a depot for the antigen (39). Ovalbumin-conjugated nanoparticles were evaluated in another study in comparison to a liquid ovalbumin formulation. They were applied in combination with a roller-type microneedle device. The IgG titers obtained in mice with the nanoparticle group were higher than that with ovalbumin solution (59).

Kumar et al. conducted a study to evaluate the combination of microneedles and nanoparticles for skin delivery of DNA vaccine. PLGA nanoparticles were coated with plasmid DNA (60). The study was successful in immunization of mice with a gene encoding a protective antigen against anthrax. Controlled release using a combination of dissolving microneedles and nanoparticles was evaluated by Demuth et al. (61). The microneedles were prepared using polyacrylic acid matrix with PLGA nanoparticles or solid PLGA at the tip. Upon insertion, the microneedles dissolved releasing the nanoparticles. The vaccine was found to be releasing from the nanoparticles over a few of weeks within the skin layers. Controlled release of vaccine from particle formulations in conjunction with microneedles was also achieved in another study conducted by Zaric et al. (62).

Combination of nanoparticles with microneedles provides a promising platform for vaccine delivery. This approach has great potential, especially with the advantages particulate formulations have such as antigen stability, depot release, and ability to enhance immune response. Further work is needed on formulation optimization and microneedle fabrication to make this into a viable option for delivering vaccines.

6.3 Conclusion

Microporation has provided an excellent platform for exploring skin as a potential route for drug administration, not limited to just small lipophilic molecules. All the published research suggests these micronscale devices have been shown to be very effective in administering a broad spectrum of drugs through skin. They can be applied to elicit local or systemic action as required. Microneedles offer endless possibilities with regard to how they can be used for drug delivery. They can be fabricated in a variety of geometries, dimensions, and compositions.

Metallic microneedles were the first type to be introduced and tested. They used materials such as silicon, titanium, and stainless steel. However, the past decade has seen the rise of dissolvable microneedles made from biodegradable materials such as sugars and polymers. Although it would seem that solid microneedles will be around for some time and have been proven effective, safety issues such as immunogenicity to the metal and creating sharp waste is worrying. Dissolvable needles do not have such issues; however, they might be subject to dosage constraints since everything needs to be incorporated into a limited space.

Microneedles also offer a few different options on the mode of delivery, so that delivery system can be tailored to the needs of the condition being addressed. A bolus dose can be achieved using coated or dissolvable microneedles that release the drug right away upon insertion into the skin. Drug solution can be injected or infused into deeper layers of the skin using hollow needles, which can also be used to sample biologic fluid such as blood to measure glucose levels. This will be a very promising approach especially in the case of diabetes. Insulin can be released from the patch based on blood glucose levels. Targeting drug to a specific depth in the skin can be achieved by altering the needle length. Controlled release is also possible. Drugs encapsulated in polymers with control-release properties can be fabricated into microneedles to obtain a desired delivery profile.

Microneedles alone have excellent features for them to be developed into a robust delivery system. This chapter has discussed studies conducted by several researchers to investigate and evaluate the potential of combining them with other technologies. A clear majority of the published studies have had a positive outcome with the combination approach. However, most of this research is in the early stages. Combining two or more techniques seems to be practical on a lab scale at this point. Existence of an FDA-approved microneedle product on the market will help boost further research in this area. Gathering more information with some sort of preclinical testing will instill confidence in these combinatorial approaches, and more thought on device design, manufacturing and scale-up, safety, and regulatory aspects is needed.

Combination of microneedles with other technologies opens up a whole new arena in the field of transdermal drug delivery. The synergistic effect seen in all the case studies discussed in this chapter showcases its potential. More research in the coming years will add value to all the efforts in pushing towards the development of a clinical product. Future studies should focus on development of prototypes and gathering preclinical data.

REFERENCES

1. Langer MRPR. Transdermal drug delivery. Nat Biotechno. 2009;26(11):1261–8.
2. Tao SL, Desai TA. Microfabricated drug delivery systems: From particles to pores. Adv Drug Deliv Rev. 2003;55:315–28.
3. Teo AL, Shearwood C, Ng KC, Lu J, Moochhala S. Transdermal microneedles for drug delivery applications. Mater Sci Eng B Solid-State Mater Adv Technol. 2006;132(1–2):151–4.
4. Prausnitz MR. Microneedles for transdermal drug delivery. Adv Drug Deliv Rev. 2004;56:581–7.
5. Arora A, Prausnitz MR, Mitragotri S. Micro-scale devices for transdermal drug delivery. Int J Pharm. 2008;364:227–36.
6. Wang Y, Thakur R, Fan Q, Michniak B. Transdermal iontophoresis: Combination strategies to improve transdermal iontophoretic drug delivery. Eur J Pharm Biopharm. 2005;60(2):179–91.
7. Polat BE, Hart D, Langer R, Blankschtein D. Ultrasound-mediated transdermal drug delivery: Mechanisms, scope, and emerging trends. , J Control Release. 2011;152:330–48.

8. Park JH, Allen MG, Prausnitz MR. Biodegradable polymer microneedles: Fabrication, mechanics and transdermal drug delivery. J Control Release. 2005;104(1):51–66.
9. Ito Y, Hagiwara E, Saeki A, Sugioka N, Takada K. Feasibility of microneedles for percutaneous absorption of insulin. Eur J Pharm Sci. 2006;29(1):82–8.
10. Li G, Badkar A, Nema S, Kolli CS, Banga AK. In vitro transdermal delivery of therapeutic antibodies using maltose microneedles. Int J Pharm. 2009;368(1–2):109–15.
11. Martanto W, Davis SP, Holiday NR, Wang J, Gill HS, Prausnitz MR. Transdermal delivery of insulin using microneedles in vivo. Pharm Res. 2004;21(6):947–52.
12. Martanto W, Moore JS, Couse T, Prausnitz MR. Mechanism of fluid infusion during microneedle insertion and retraction. J Control Release. 2006;112(3):357–61.
13. Davidson A, Al-Qallaf B, Das DB. Transdermal drug delivery by coated microneedles: Geometry effects on effective skin thickness and drug permeability. Chem Eng Res Des. 2008;86(11):1196–206.
14. Verbaan FJ, Bal SM, van den Berg DJ, Dijksman JA, van Hecke M, Verpoorten H, et al. Improved piercing of microneedle arrays in dermatomed human skin by an impact insertion method. J Control Release. 2008;128(1):80–8.
15. Kalia YN, Naik A, Garrison J, Guy RH. Iontophoretic drug delivery. Adv Drug Deliv Rev. 2004;56: 619–58.
16. Green PG. Iontophoretic delivery of peptide drugs. J Control Release. 1996;41(1–2):33–48.
17. Pikal MJ. The role of electroosmotic flow in transdermal iontophoresis. Adv Drug Deliv Rev. 2001;46:281–305.
18. Cázares-Delgadillo J, Naik A, Ganem-Rondero A, Quintanar-Guerrero D, Kalia YN. Transdermal delivery of cytochrome C—A 12.4 kDa protein—Across intact skin by constant-current iontophoresis. Pharm Res. 2007;24(7):1360–8.
19. Wu XM, Todo H, Sugibayashi K. Enhancement of skin permeation of high molecular compounds by a combination of microneedle pretreatment and iontophoresis. J Control Release. 2007;118(2):189–95.
20. Vemulapalli V, Bai Y, Kalluri H, Herwadkar A, Kim H, Davis SP, et al. In vivo iontophoretic delivery of salmon calcitonin across microporated skin. J Pharm Sci. 2012;101(8):2861–9.
21. Vemulapalli V, Yang Y, Friden PM, Banga AK. Synergistic effect of iontophoresis and soluble microneedles for transdermal delivery of methotrexate. J Pharm Pharmacol [Internet]. 2008;60(1): 27–33. Available from: http://doi.wiley.com/10.1211/jpp.60.1.0004
22. Katikaneni S, Badkar A, Nema S, Banga AK. Molecular charge mediated transport of a 13 kD protein across microporated skin. Int J Pharm. 2009;378(1–2):93–100.
23. Lin W, Cormier M, Samiee A, Griffin A, Johnson B, Teng CL, et al. Transdermal delivery of antisense oligonucleotides with microprojection patch (Macroflux®) technology. Pharm Res. 2001;18(12):1789–93.
24. Lanke SSS, Kolli CS, Strom JG, Banga AK. Enhanced transdermal delivery of low molecular weight heparin by barrier perturbation. Int J Pharm. 2009;365(1):26–33.
25. Katikaneni S, Li G, Badkar A, Banga AK. Transdermal delivery of a approximately 13 kDa protein— an in vivo comparison of physical enhancement methods. J Drug Target [Internet]. 2010;18(2):141–7. Available from: http://www.ncbi.nlm.nih.gov/pubmed/19772395
26. Mitragotri S, Kost J. Low-frequency sonophoresis: A review. Adv Drug Deliv Rev. 2004;56:589–601.
27. Nyborg WL, Carson PL, Carstensen EL, Dunn F, Miller DL, Miller MW, et al. Exposure criteria for medical diagnostic ultrasound: II. Criteria based on all known mechanisms [Internet]. NCRP Report. 2002. i-ix+1-545. Available from: http://www.embase.com/search/results?subaction=view record&from=export&id=L36410282%5Cnhttp://sfx.aub.aau.dk/sfxaub?sid=EMBASE&issn=008 3209X&id=doi:&atitle=Exposure+criteria+for+medical+diagnostic+ultrasound%3A+II.+Criteria+ based+on+all+known+mechanisms&st
28. Chen B, Wei J, Iliescu C. Sonophoretic enhanced microneedles array (SEMA)-Improving the efficiency of transdermal drug delivery. Sensors Actuators, B Chem. 2010;145(1):54–60.
29. Han T, Das DB. Permeability enhancement for transdermal delivery of large molecule using low-frequency sonophoresis combined with microneedles. J Pharm Sci. 2013;102(10):3614–22.
30. Han T, Das DB. Potential of combined ultrasound and microneedles for enhanced transdermal drug permeation: A review. , Eur J Pharm Biopharm. 2015;89:312–28.
31. Ita K. Perspectives on transdermal electroporation. Pharmaceutics. 2016;8(1).
32. Naik A, Kalia YN, Guy RH. Transdermal drug delivery: Overcoming the skin's barrier function., Pharm Sci Technol Today. 2000;3:318–26.

33. Kumar R, Philip A. Modified Transdermal Technologies: Breaking the Barriers of Drug Permeation via the Skin. Trop J Pharm Res [Internet]. 2007;6(1):633–44. Available from: http://www.ajol.info/index. php/tjpr/article/view/14641

34. Wilke N, Hibert C, O'Brien J, Morrissey A. Silicon microneedle electrode array with temperature monitoring for electroporation. Sensor Actuat A-Phys. 2005;123–124:319–25.

35. Hooper JW, Golden JW, Ferro AM, King AD. Smallpox DNA vaccine delivered by novel skin electroporation device protects mice against intranasal poxvirus challenge. Vaccine. 2007;25(10):1814–23.

36. Yan K, Todo H, Sugibayashi K. Transdermal drug delivery by in-skin electroporation using a microneedle array. Int J Pharm. 2010;397(1–2):77–83.

37. Prow TW, Grice JE, Lin LL, Faye R, Butler M, Becker W, et al. Nanoparticles and microparticles for skin drug delivery. Adv Drug Deliv Rev. 2011;63:470–91.

38. Patravale V, Dandekar P, Jain R. Nanoparticulate drug delivery: Perspectives on the transition from laboratory to market [Internet]. 2012;1–229. Available from: http://www.scopus.com/inward/record. url?eid=2-s2.0-84903652152&partnerID=40&md5=2d9cddfc744ae4ea56f06554e7c3114a

39. Donnelly RF, Singh TRR, Morrow DIJ, Woolfson AD. Microneedle-mediated transdermal and intradermal drug delivery. 2012.

40. Agüeros M, Espuelas S, Esparza I, Calleja P, Peñuelas I, Ponchel G, et al. Cyclodextrin-poly(anhydride) nanoparticles as new vehicles for oral drug delivery. Expert Opin Drug Deliv [Internet]. 2011;8(6): 721–34. Available from: http://dx.doi.org/10.1517/17425247.2011.572069%5Cnhttp://informahealthcare. com/doi/pdfplus/10.1517/17425247.2011.572069

41. Ponchel G, Irache JM. Specific and non-specific bioadhesive particulate systems for oral delivery to the gastrointestinal tract. Adv Drug Deliv Rev. 1998;34:191–219.

42. Nava-Arzaluz MG, Calderon-Lojero I, Quintanar-Guerrero D, Villalobos-Garcia R, Ganem-Quintanar A. Microneedles as transdermal delivery systems: Combination with other enhancing strategies. Curr Drug Deliv [Internet]. 2012;9(1):57–73. Available from: http://www.eurekaselect.com/openurl/content. php?genre=article&issn=1567-2018&volume=9&issue=1&spage=57

43. McAllister DV, Wang PM, Davis SP, Park J-H, Canatella PJ, Allen MG, et al. Microfabricated needles for transdermal delivery of macromolecules and nanoparticles: Fabrication methods and transport studies. Proc Natl Acad Sci [Internet]. 2003;100(24):13755–60. Available from: http://www.pnas.org/cgi/ doi/10.1073/pnas.2331316100

44. Coulman SA, Barrow D, Anstey A, Gateley C, Morrissey A, Wilke N, et al. Minimally invasive cutaneous delivery of macromolecules and plasmid DNA via microneedles. Curr Drug Deliv. 2006;3(1):65–75.

45. Chabri F, Bouris K, Jones T, Barrow D, Hann A, Allender C, et al. Microfabricated silicon microneedles for nonviral cutaneous gene delivery. Br J Dermatol. 2004;150(5):869–77.

46. Pearton M, Allender C, Brain K, Anstey A, Gateley C, Wilke N, et al. Gene delivery to the epidermal cells of human skin explants using microfabricated microneedles and hydrogel formulations. Pharm Res. 2008;25(2):407–16.

47. Zhang W, Gao J, Zhu Q, Zhang M, Ding X, Wang X, et al. Penetration and distribution of PLGA nanoparticles in the human skin treated with microneedles. Int J Pharm. 2010;402(1–2):205–12.

48. Gomaa YA, Garland MJ, McInnes FJ, Donnelly RF, El-Khordagui LK, Wilson CG. Microneedle/ nanoencapsulation-mediated transdermal delivery: Mechanistic insights. Eur J Pharm Biopharm. 2014;86(2):145–55.

49. Wang PM, Cornwell M, Hill J, Prausnitz MR. Precise microinjection into skin using hollow microneedles. J Invest Dermatol. 2006;126(5):1080–7.

50. Häfeli UO, Mokhtari A, Liepmann D, Stoeber B. In vivo evaluation of a microneedle-based miniature syringe for intradermal drug delivery. Biomed Microdevices. 2009;11(5):943–50.

51. Ito Y, Hagiwara E, Saeki A, Sugioka N, Takada K. Sustained-release self-dissolving micropiles for percutaneous absorption of insulin in mice. J Drug Target. 2007;15(5):323–6.

52. Chen H, Zhu H, Zheng J, Mou D, Wan J, Zhang J, et al. Iontophoresis-driven penetration of nanovesicles through microneedle-induced skin microchannels for enhancing transdermal delivery of insulin. J Control Release. 2009;139(1):63–72.

53. Yu J, Zhang Y, Ye Y, DiSanto R, Sun W, Ranson D, et al. Microneedle-array patches loaded with hypoxia-sensitive vesicles provide fast glucose-responsive insulin delivery. Proc Natl Acad Sci [Internet]. 2015;112(27):8260–5. Available from: http://www.pnas.org/lookup/doi/10.1073/pnas.1505405112

54. Storni T, Kündig TM, Senti G, Johansen P. Immunity in response to particulate antigen-delivery systems. Adv Drug Deliv Rev. 2005;57:333–55.

55. Gutierro I, Hernández RM, Igartua M, Gascón AR, Pedraz JL. Size dependent immune response after subcutaneous, oral and intranasal administration of BSA loaded nanospheres. Vaccine. 2002;21(1–2):67–77.

56. Jaganathan KS, Vyas SP. Strong systemic and mucosal immune responses to surface-modified PLGA microspheres containing recombinant Hepatitis B antigen administered intranasally. Vaccine. 2006;24(19):4201–11.

57. Mahapatro A, Singh DK. Biodegradable nanoparticles are excellent vehicle for site directed in-vivo delivery of drugs and vaccines. J Nanobiotechnology [Internet]. 2011;9(1):55. Available from: http://jnanobiotechnology.biomedcentral.com/articles/10.1186/1477-3155-9-55

58. De Geest BG, Willart MA, Hammad H, Lambrecht BN, Pollard C, Bogaert P, et al. Polymeric multilayer capsule-mediated vaccination induces protective immunity against cancer and viral infection. ACS Nano. 2012;6(3):2136–49.

59. Kumar A, Li X, Sandoval MA, Rodriguez BL, Sloat BR, Cui Z. Permeation of antigen protein-conjugated nanoparticles and live bacteria through microneedle-treated mouse skin. Int J Nanomedicine. 2011;6:1253–64.

60. Kumar A, Wonganan P, Sandoval MA, Li X, Zhu S, Cui Z. Microneedle-mediated transcutaneous immunization with plasmid DNA coated on cationic PLGA nanoparticles. J Control Release. 2012;163(2):230–9.

61. Demuth PC, Garcia-Beltran WF, Ai-Ling ML, Hammond PT, Irvine DJ. Composite dissolving microneedles for coordinated control of antigen and adjuvant delivery kinetics in transcutaneous vaccination. Adv Funct Mater. 2013;23(2):161–72.

62. Zaric M, Lyubomska O, Touzelet O, Poux C, Al-Zahrani S, Fay F, et al. Skin dendritic cell targeting via microneedle arrays laden with antigen-encapsulated poly- D, l -Lactide- Co -Glycolide nanoparticles induces efficient antitumor and antiviral immune responses. ACS Nano. 2013;7(3):2042–55.

7

Medical Applications of Microneedles

Samantha Tran
Stryker School of Medicine, Western Michigan University

Raja Sivamani
Department of Dermatology, University of California-Davis
Pacific Skin Institute

Microneedling is a minimally invasive procedure that creates small pores called microchannels in the stratum corneum of the epidermis layer of the skin. The microneedles can extend down farther and create microchannels that reach the dermis layer of the skin, while keeping the skin partially intact.[1] By creating these microchannels, microneedles increase the skin's permeability and enhance the absorption of topically applied medications and therapies.

7.1 Types of Microneedles

Microneedles can be made from a variety of materials including silicon, metal, polymers, ceramic, and silica glass.[2,3] There are three general classes of microneedles: (1) solid, (2) dissolvable, and (3) hollow-bore.

Solid microneedles: These create the microchannels in the epidermis to enhance delivery of topical drugs (e.g., via a drug-loaded patch, or a gel, cream, or ointment) so that the drugs can effectively penetrate the skin. The needles might be either uncoated or coated with a drug of interest, so that, as they penetrate, the drug is immediately delivered.[3] Most clinical studies have utilized the use of solid microneedles to create temporary holes through which topical medications are applied.

Dissolvable microneedles: These will naturally dissolve and release the drug when the needle is embedded into the skin and the tip comes in contact with the interstitial fluid.[3] The few studies that have utilized dissolving microneedles in a clinical setting have been limited to vaccination studies (Figure 7.1).

Hollow-bore microneedles: These have openings at either the tip or the sides that allow a drug to be delivered through the central lumen into the skin. The main limitations of hollow-bore microneedles are the potential for clogging of the opening with tissue during insertion and flow resistance due to compression of the dermal tissue around the tips.[3] The few studies that have utilized hollow-bore microneedles have been largely limited to vaccination-based studies.

7.2 Microneedle Length

Microneedles come in a variety of lengths depending on what treatment is needed.

Use	Microneedle Length	Mechanism
Topical drug application	~0.7 mm or less	Creates small pores so that drugs can effectively penetrate the skin. Typically used for transdermal penetration enhancement.
Aging and/or wrinkles	~0.5 to 1.0 mm	Induces collagen formation and skin remodeling.
Acne scars or hypertrophic scars	~1.5 to 2.0 mm	Destroys the scar collagen bundles.

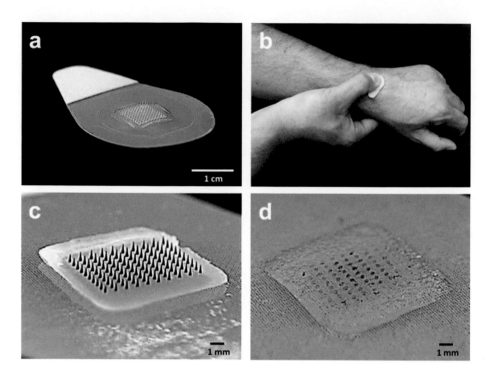

FIGURE 7.1 Microneedle patch (MNP) for influenza vaccination. **(a)** The MNP contains an array of 100 microneedles measuring 650 µm tall mounted on an adhesive backing. **(b)** The MNP is manually administered to the wrist, enabling self-administration by study subjects. **(c)** Microneedles encapsulate influenza vaccine (represented here by blue dye) within a water-soluble matrix. **(d)** After application to the skin, the needles dissolve, depositing vaccine and leaving behind a patch backing that can be discarded as non-sharp waste. (From ref. 7 with permission.)

In general, only a superficial penetration of the epidermis is needed for drug delivery, while a deeper penetration into the dermis is required for cosmetic treatments for scars and acne.[4]

The length of the microneedle also impacts the time interval between each treatment. Longer needles necessitate a longer gap between treatments to allow the skin to heal properly.[4]

7.3 Medical Therapies

Microneedles are an innovative device that can be used to deliver vaccine and enhance transdermal drug delivery.[5]

7.3.1 Vaccinations

The benefit of a transdermal vaccine is that it can create a more robust antibody response compared to an intramuscular vaccine. One of the touted benefits of microneedle-based vaccination is the possibility of painless vaccinations.

One clinical pilot study compared intramuscular injection and microneedle-based injection with a 600-micron array of microneedles of influenza vaccines. The study was conducted in six treatment arms among 370 volunteers.[6] Microneedle-based injections generated sufficient immunogenicity and less pain with the injection than the intramuscular injection, but caused more local edema and redness.

Another pilot phase 1 randomized study of 100 participants compared conventional administration of influenza vaccines through intramuscular injection with self-administration of dissolving microneedles (650 microns in a water-based dissolving matrix).[7] The investigators found that microneedle-based injections were just as effective at creating antigenicity while the reported pain was lower than for intramuscular injections. While pain-related side effects were lower, the two modes of injection had similar side effects of local redness and fatigue.

7.3.2 Topical Anesthesia

Microneedles-based drug delivery has also been tested for enhancement of topical anesthesia. A study of 15 participants that utilized 500 micron glass-based hollow microneedles found that microneedle-based injections were just as effective as hypodermic needle–based injections for lidocaine.[8] The study found that 80% of participants did not consider the microneedle-based injection painful and 77% of participants preferred the microneedle-based approach to anesthesia. Another study evaluated the use of solid microneedle (200 microns) pretreatment followed by topical anesthesia in 21 participants and the treatments were randomized to each forearm. One arm received the microneedle pretreatment while the other received sham microneedle pretreatment prior to application of topical 4% lidocaine cream.[9] The microneedle-treated arm was significantly less sensitive to needle lancet pain stimulation at 30 min, and it showed improved pain tolerance with those with higher baseline pain by 10 min.

7.3.3 Photodynamic Therapy

Photodynamic therapy is typically used in the treatment of actinic keratoses and depends upon topical application of 5-aminolevulinic acid that is allowed to incubate for an hour and then the skin is exposed to blue light for the therapy. Two studies evaluated how microneedle pretreatment may alter the incubation times needed with the 5-aminolevulinic acid. The first study utilized 690-micron solid microneedles that were stamped onto the face as a pretreatment prior to topical application of the 5-aminolevulinic acid.[10] The study utilized a split-face design in 48 participants to compare the standard 60-min incubation on the sham-treated side versus a 20-, 40-, or 60-min incubation (randomized) on the microneedle-treated side. The investigators found that a 20-min incubation on the microneedle-pretreated side was as effective at clearing actinic keratoses as the standard 60-min incubation (Figure 7.2). A follow-up study in 33 participants evaluated the role of using 500-micron solid microneedle pretreatments versus sham microneedle pretreatment in a split-faced design that compared lower incubations times with the 5-aminolevulinic acid in a head-to-head fashion at 10 min and 20 min.[11] While there was not statistical difference between the microneedle and sham-treated sides with the 10-min incubation, there was a statistically significant improvement on the microneedle-treated side at 20 min of incubation (76% on microneedle side versus 58% on the sham side, $p < .01$). The two studies suggest that microneedle pretreatment can enhance the transcutaneous penetration of 5-aminolevulinic acid and may allow for reduction of incubation times from 60 to 20 min. The results warrant further study in an expanded group of participants to assess the role of microneedle pretreatment.

7.3.4 Glucose Sampling

Aside from delivering drugs, microneedles can be used as sensors for diagnostic purposes. For example, microneedles can take a very small sample of blood and sample the glucose concentration in patients with diabetes.[12] Compared to the current glucometer with lancets, the microneedle will provide a painless option to monitor glucose levels. By making glucose monitoring simpler, we can increase patients' compliance and ability to control the sugars, improving health outcomes for them. A pilot clinical study in 10 diabetic subjects showed that glucose sampling was both accurate and well tolerated over a 72-h period. Longer use of microneedle sampling devices will need to be assessed in future studies for long-term usability and tolerability.

7.4 Possible Side Effects and Risks

Overall, microneedles are well tolerated. Because it is minimally invasive and the epidermis is not broken, there is a lower risk of infection, post-inflammatory hyperpigmentation, and scarring.[1] Furthermore, the microchannels created by the needles close within 60–90 min, which reduces the risk of infections.

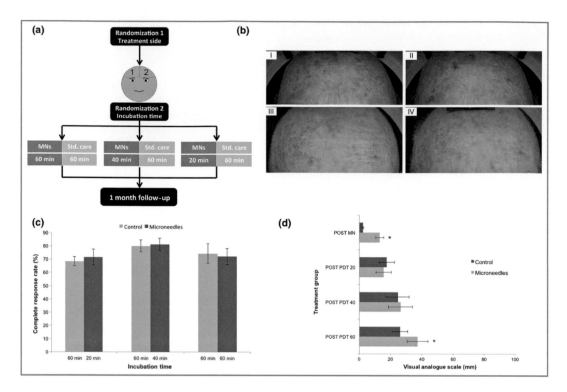

FIGURE 7.2 **(a)** Study flow schematic. **(b)** Forehead view of actinic keratoses before (I and III) and 1 month after (II and IV) photodynamic therapy (PDT) treatment with microneedle (MN) pretreatment (left forehead in all images) and with sham pretreatment (right forehead in all images). **(c)** Actinic keratosis complete response rate (CRR) results. Average CRR (SEM) for the 20-, 40-, and 60-min treatment and control arms were 71.4% (5.8) and 68.3% (3.3); 81.1% (4.6) and 79.9% (4.5); and 72.1% (5.5) and 74.2% (6.9) respectively ($n = 15$, $P = 0.51$; $n = 16$, $P = 0.79$; $n = 16$, $P = 0.72$). **(d)** Pain scoring after MN application. Pain assessment using a 100-mm visual analogue scale was performed after MN pretreatment and after PDT in all treatment groups (PDT 20, 20-min aminolaevulinic acid [ALA] incubation; PDT 40, 40-min ALA incubation; PDT 60, 60-min ALA incubation). Average pain scores after MN pretreatment (SEM) in the treatment and control arms were 13.1 mm (2.6) and 2.4 mm (0.5) respectively ($N = 48$, $P < 0.01$). Average pain scores after PDT light treatment (SEM) in the 20-, 40-, and 60-min treatment and control arms were 15.7 mm (4.9) and 17.7 mm (4.9); 26.4 mm (7.5) and 24.7 mm (7.1); and 37.2 mm (6.6) and 26.0 mm (4.9) respectively ($n = 15$, $P = 0.35$; $n = 16$, $P = 0.23$; $n = 17$, $P = 0.046$). *$P < 0.05$, **$P < 0.01$. (From ref. 10 with permission.)

Side effects are minimal and include transient redness, mild dryness, and small hematomas.[13] Erythema may be present after treatment lasting up to three days, although this may persist longer with vaccinations as the vaccine may induce redness apart from the microneedle itself.

Finally, it will be important to carefully choose what substances are delivered transcutaneously, as there is always the potential for an allergy to topically applied products. As clinical research expands in the area of microneedle-assisted topical delivery, we will get an increasingly better understanding of its clinical efficacy and side effects.

REFERENCES

1. Hogan S, Velez MW, Ibrahim O. Microneedling: a new approach for treating textural abnormalities and scars. *Semin Cutan Med Surg.* 2017;36(4):155–163.
2. Bhatnagar S, Dave K, Venuganti VVK. Microneedles in the clinic. *J Control Release.* 2017;260:164–182.
3. Garland MJ, Migalska K, Mahmood TM, Singh TR, Woolfson AD, Donnelly RF. Microneedle arrays as medical devices for enhanced transdermal drug delivery. *Expert Rev Med Devices.* 2011;8(4):459–482.
4. Singh A, Yadav S. Microneedling: advances and widening horizons. *Indian Dermatol Online J.* 2016;7(4):244–254.

5. Kwon KM, Lim SM, Choi S, et al. Microneedles: quick and easy delivery methods of vaccines. *Clin Exp Vaccine Res.* 2017;6(2):156–159.

6. Levin Y, Kochba E, Shukarev G, Rusch S, Herrera-Taracena G, van Damme P. A phase 1, open-label, randomized study to compare the immunogenicity and safety of different administration routes and doses of virosomal influenza vaccine in elderly. *Vaccine.* 2016;34(44):5262–5272.

7. Rouphael NG, Paine M, Mosley R, et al. The safety, immunogenicity, and acceptability of inactivated influenza vaccine delivered by microneedle patch (TIV-MNP 2015): a randomised, partly blinded, placebo-controlled, phase 1 trial. *Lancet.* 2017;390(10095):649–658.

8. Gupta J, Denson DD, Felner EI, Prausnitz MR. Rapid local anesthesia in humans using minimally invasive microneedles. *Clin J Pain.* 2012;28(2):129–135.

9. Ornelas J, Foolad N, Shi V, Burney W, Sivamani RK. Effect of microneedle pretreatment on topical anesthesia: a randomized clinical trial. *JAMA Dermatol.* 2016;152(4):476–477.

10. Lev-Tov H, Larsen L, Zackria R, Chahal H, Eisen DB, Sivamani RK. Microneedle-assisted incubation during aminolaevulinic acid photodynamic therapy of actinic keratoses: a randomized controlled evaluator-blind trial. *Br J Dermatol.* 2017;176(2):543–545.

11. Petukhova TA, Hassoun LA, Foolad N, Barath M, Sivamani RK. Effect of expedited microneedle-assisted photodynamic therapy for field treatment of actinic keratoses: a randomized clinical trial. *JAMA Dermatol.* 2017;153(7):637–643.

12. Smart WH, Subramanian K. The use of silicon microfabrication technology in painless blood glucose monitoring. *Diabetes Technol Ther.* 2000;2(4):549–559.

13. Al Qarqaz F, Al-Yousef A. Skin microneedling for acne scars associated with pigmentation in patients with dark skin. *J Cosmet Dermatol.* 2018;17(3):390–395.

8

Therapeutic Drug and Biomolecule Monitoring Potential for Microneedle Technologies

Sahan A. Ranamukhaarachchi[1,2], Urs O. Häfeli[2,3]
[1] *Department of Electrical and Computer Engineering, University of British Columbia*
[2] *Faculty of Pharmaceutical Sciences, University of British Columbia*
[3] *Department of Pharmacy, University of Copenhagen*

8.1 Introduction

Therapeutic drug and biomolecule monitoring (TDM) is the process of measuring the concentration of active pharmaceutical compounds and biomolecules in blood that, with proper interpretation, will influence therapy and future medical procedures [1]. TDM is of utmost importance when drug candidates with a narrow therapeutic window are administered (Figure 8.1). Outside of this window, a patient can be overdosed to cause potentially life-threatening side effects or underdosed to provide ineffective therapy [2]. Similarly, there are biomolecules that become available or change concentration in the blood after intake of food and beverages, such as glucose, that are not therapeutic drugs, but rather metabolites or disease-causing agents that need to be monitored. The ability of continuously monitoring such biomolecules provides information for timely and effective treatment to ensure the health and well-being of patients [3]. Furthermore, the detection of elevated levels of specific markers, such as nitric oxide for inflammatory diseases or the protein CA19-9 for pancreatic cancer, can indicate the occurrence of physiological changes in the human body. Monitoring such biomolecules thus will help to diagnose health issues early and start treatment on time [4–6].

TDM and diagnostic testing are conventionally conducted in blood samples withdrawn from patients at regular intervals [7]. Blood sampling utilizes an invasive needle, or another sharp device such as a lancet, to access blood and extract it from capillaries or veins. Each TDM time point requires at least 100 μL of whole blood [8]. Whole blood requires processing, such as centrifugation to extract serum, before the analysis can be performed. Many of the TDM analytes in blood are separated and quantified using expensive and time-consuming laboratory processes that include liquid chromatography and mass spectrometry (e.g., LCMS) [7]. Significant resources are thus allocated to TDM analyses in terms of money and time, and there exist substantial opportunities to monitor and diagnose patients in more efficient ways.

An exciting opportunity to improve on the painful blood sampling and expensive and slow sample processing in TDM is the exploration of interstitial fluid (ISF) as a matrix for biosensing of drugs and biomolecules, many of which show a predictable correlation with blood concentrations. With the development of technologies that allow easy, minimally invasive, and pain-free access to ISF, novel concepts have begun to emerge that will lead to a paradigm shift in TDM and point-of-care diagnostics. The objectives of this chapter are to (1) explore the potential for TDM in ISF and compare it to blood analyses and (2) provide a review of the significant work completed to date using microneedle (MN) technologies for biosensing in TDM applications.

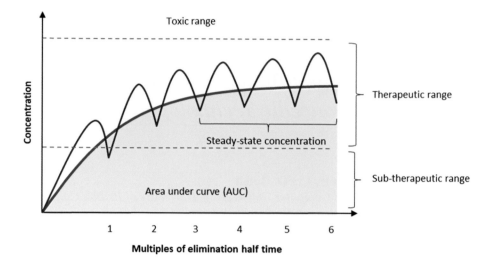

FIGURE 8.1 A typical therapeutic drug monitoring profile showing the narrow therapeutic window. The red line indicates the blood concentration profile of the drug during multiple dosing; the ideally provided blood concentration required for therapy is shown in blue. The total dose delivered by the blue curve, shown as the light blue area, is called the area under the curve (AUC). (Figure obtained from Kim *et al.* (2008) with modifications [2].)

8.2 Therapeutically Monitored Drugs

Clinically, about a dozen drugs are regularly tested in patients to verify that the drug's blood concentration is in the optimal range, which means non-toxic but effective. The most important TDM drugs include the immunosuppressant drugs tacrolimus and mycophenolate, the antibiotics gentamicin and vancomycin, and some antiepileptic and anticancer drugs (Table 8.1).

TABLE 8.1

Clinically Important TDM Drugs

Drug Category	Drug	Frequency of Use
Immunosuppressants to prevent rejection of transplanted organs, autoimmune disorders	Cyclosporine Mycophenolate*, tacrolimus, sirolimus	Trough or 2 h post dose Trough
Antibiotics for treatment of resistant bacteria	Aminoglycosides (amikacin, gentamicin, tobramycin), vancomycin*	Both trough and 1 h post dose (daily)
Cardiac drugs for congestive heart failure, arrhythmias, angina	Digoxin, digitoxin Amiodarone Lidocaine, procainamide	Trough or > 6 h post dose Trough 2 h post dose
Antiepileptic drugs to prevent seizures	Carbamazepine, levetiracetam, valproic acid Phenobarbital*, phenytoin	Trough (daily) At steady state (weekly or longer)
Bronchodilators for asthma treatment	Theophylline*	Trough and 2 h (immediate release) or 4–8 h (slow release) post dose
Anticancer drugs, also used in psoriasis and rheumatoid arthritis	Methotrexate*	Often 24, 48, and 72 h after high-dose therapy
Psychiatric drugs for bipolar disorder and psychosis	Lithium Valproic acid, amitriptyline, clozapine, fluoxetine	12 h post-dose Trough

*Suitable or likely suitable for direct concentration measurements in ISF [10]
Adapted from Hallworth and Watson [9].

Testing the drug concentrations instead of blood in ISF would be directly possible in vancomycin and other drugs listed in Table 8.1. Others, such as tacrolimus, are not appropriate for these analyses, as they are typically highly protein-bound and cannot be found in ISF or do not establish a reliable presence there with known correlations to blood concentrations and drug effects. Correlations between blood and ISF concentrations of a few important TDM drugs have been established recently [11], but more work is necessary to turn the currently exotic method into a useful and practical method.

For suitable drugs, however, the benefits of ISF sampling and especially on-device analysis can be major. Microneedle sampling of ISF is pain-free and without bleeding, so even older people with sensitive skin and children of all ages could undergo extensive analyses. One example in which ISF sampling would have huge benefits is the measuring of the mycophenolate pharmacokinetics in pediatric intestinal transplantation patients [12]. Children show enormous differences in the rate of mycophenolate metabolism. Jia *et al.* (2017) showed, for example, that the AUC of three children after taking enterocoated mycophenolate sodium was 5.3, 56.5, and 87.5 mg h L^{-1}, which is an interindividual difference of 16 times. Since side effects are often serious and include headache, nausea, and bloody diarrhea, it is important to establish a patient's reached drug concentration. Currently, this requires typically 11 blood samplings within 12 hours, something that is difficult to do in a child, and would be easy to accomplish with ISF sampling using microneedles.

8.3 Microneedle Technologies for Therapeutic Drug Monitoring

MN technologies have been developed, prototyped, and evaluated *in vitro* and *in vivo* for their respective TDM, diagnostics, and physiological health monitoring, as described in this section. Work performed to date has explored many strategies to employ MN devices for minimally invasive diagnostics and monitoring activities creatively and uniquely. These strategies include point-of-care diagnostics devices, using: MNs for ISF extraction followed by off-device analysis, ISF extraction followed by on-device analysis without ISF extraction at all; and continuous monitoring systems using MNs. As the area of MN-integrated biosensors for TDM and diagnostics improve and continue to develop, it is likely that more unique and creative approaches will emerge to change the ways current TDM procedures are conducted.

8.3.1 Interstitial Fluid Extraction Devices for Off-Device Analysis

ISF, which is abundant in the skin layers, is tightly trapped in its extracellular matrices [13], presenting challenges to successful and repeatable extraction for biosensing applications. Considering that ISF is present at ~20 nL mm^{-2} in the epidermis and ~800 nL mm^{-2} in the dermis [13], the necessity for extraction of large volumes of ISF for quantitative biomolecule analyses appears to be a major roadblock in developing biosensors for ISF extraction. However, several studies have successfully demonstrated various techniques for ISF extraction from the skin, followed by analysis of its content outside the ISF-collecting MN device (termed *off-device analysis* henceforth).

In one of the first studies exploring the potential of ISF extraction using MNs, Wang *et al.* (2005) used a glass MN device to penetrate 0.7–1.5 mm into the skin in hairless rats and healthy adults, and collect ISF using a 26.6–66.6 kPa vacuum for 2–10 min [14]. They collected 1–10 μL of ISF and measured ISF glucose concentrations, and compared to blood glucose collected from the tail vein of rats and finger sticks in humans. ISF glucose levels correlated well with blood glucose levels in rats and human subjects, although a 20-min time lag was observed. Several practical challenges faced during implementation of this method included multiple steps required to conduct the analysis, requirement of transferring the fluid out of the collection device for analysis, and evaporation of the collected fluid leading to measurement variability and error. Nonetheless, Wang *et al.* provided the first indication of ISF extraction through pores created through MNs on the skin.

To obviate the need for vacuum-assisted extraction of fluid and risk of ISF evaporation, Sakaguchi *et al.* (2012) developed an alternative approach to poke-and-collect [15]. Sakaguchi *et al.* utilized solid MN arrays to create micropores on the skin surface of human subjects through an applicator-driven insertion. Upon removal of the MN arrays, a hydrogel patch was placed on the MN-treated area of the skin to facilitate the collection of ISF from the skin by swelling action. Glucose and sodium ion concentrations were determined from the hydrogel matrix to generate the AUC for ISF (as shown in Figure 8.1), and compare to plasma glucose from the oral glucose tolerance test (OGTT). Sakaguchi *et al.* found strong correlations between the ISF and plasma glucose levels, providing a simple solution for glucose measurements without requiring blood. While they could extract and assess multiple analytes from ISF through one process, drawbacks of the proposed process included prolonged measurement time compared to the standard measurement, many steps required to obtain a measurement, and variability in the rate of fluid collection during sampling.

Combining the approaches used by Sakaguchi *et al.*, Donnelly *et al.* (2014) developed a hydrogel-forming MN array, which increased its mass upon skin insertion, due to uptake of ISF from the skin by the hydrogel [16]. These MNs were fabricated using blends of hydrolyzed poly(methyl vinylether-co-maleic anhydride) and polyethylene glycol (PEG) cross-linked by esterification. Initially, it was shown that the mass of the MN array increased by 30% after 6 h of being inserted in the skin. In a subsequent study, Caffarrel-Salvador *et al.* (2015) demonstrated ISF extraction by swelling action of these hydrogel-forming MNs during insertion for 1–2 h *ex vivo* into excised porcine skin, and *in vivo* into rats and human subjects (Figure 8.2) [17]. Theophylline and caffeine were extracted from the hydrogel MNs and assessed using high-performance liquid chromatography (HPLC), while glucose concentration was determined using a glucose assay kit.

In a similar study, Romanyuk *et al.* (2014) developed solid MN patches with cross-linked hydrogels composed of poly(methyl vinylether-alt-maleic acid) and PEG, and demonstrated ISF uptakes up to

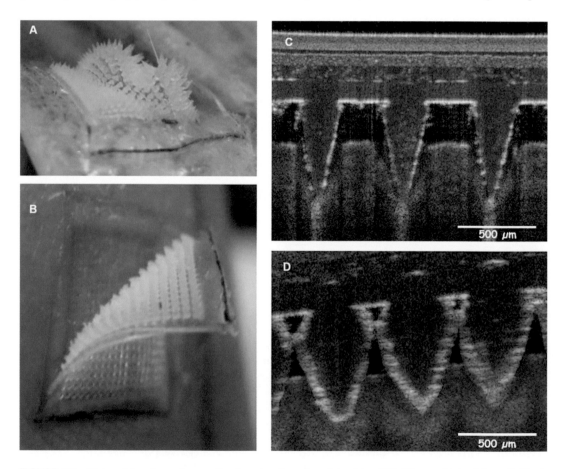

FIGURE 8.2 Hydrogel-forming microneedles for extraction of analytes from ISF. (Figure obtained from Caffarel-Salvador *et al.* (2015) with permission [17].)

50 times the original array volume [18]. These patches were manually inserted by pressing into rat skin in vivo for 1 h to extract ISF, followed by wetting the MN patch with 0.1 mL of water and ultracentrifugation to extract the collected ISF from the hydrogel matrix. Though the ability to extract ISF was demonstrated through hydrogel-forming MN arrays, major limitations needed to be overcome for these devices to be commercially viable, including but not limited to prolonged ISF collection periods, a need to extract the ISF and its content from the hydrogel matrix, the requirement of large volumes (microliter-range) of ISF for sample evaluation, and the requirement for large and expensive laboratory equipment to conduct measurements.

8.3.2 Interstitial Fluid Extraction for On-Device Analysis

Due to the limited volume of ISF that could be extracted from the skin, MN-integrated biosensing systems were developed to extract ISF and perform the biomolecule analysis on-device, without being transferred to a separate instrument. In most on-device examples, the collected ISF is transferred out of the MNs to a different compartment of the same biosensing system, such as a fluid reservoir or a sensing chamber.

In the earliest demonstration of the capability of ISF extraction using MNs, Mukerjee *et al.* (2004) designed an integrated biosensing system with a hollow MN array for transdermal biological fluid extraction and sample analysis, all in one integrated device [19]. Hollow silicon MN arrays were fabricated using a combination of deep reactive ion etching (DRIE), diamond-blade circular sawing, and wet chemical etching techniques. The MN lumens were connected to a microfluidic chip located at the back side of the array, where continuation of the MN lumens to microfluidic channels ensured the flow of fluid by capillary action to the desired location in the chip. Mukerjee *et al.* demonstrated the ability of the system to collect non-biological and biological fluids, such as water, glycerol, ISF, and whole blood using this system. They demonstrated the ability of their hollow MN system with a "snake fang" tip design to extract ISF in vivo from human earlobe skin over a 15–20 min period. The extracted ISF was analyzed qualitatively for glucose by placing components of a commercial blood glucose test strip on the fluid reservoir behind the MN array in the chip, and observing a color change in the test strip that indicated a glucose concentration between 80–120 mg dL^{-1}. The drawbacks of the Mukerjee sensor were the needs for microliter-level volumes of ISF for analysis, prolonged time to collect ISF, and transfer of ISF to the back side of the MN for analysis.

In a similar, but potentially more advanced approach for glucose sensing, Zimmerman *et al.* (2004) developed a hollow silicon MN array to be integrated into an enzymatic glucose sensor with a porous dialysis membrane [20]. Using this glucose sensor, Zimmerman *et al.* demonstrated a significant sensor response after exposure to ISF suggesting the capability and potential for glucose sensing.

A decade later, Strambini *et al.* (2015) developed a similar glucose-sensing MN device with hollow silicon dioxide MN arrays, containing projections at 100-μm height, 4-μm tip diameter, and 1×10^6 needles cm^{-2} [21]. These MN projections were an order of magnitude smaller than other MN technologies that have been used for biosensing. A 10-μL-volume reservoir on a chip is integrated to the back side of the MN array for ISF collection via capillary action through the MN lumens. A screen-printed enzymatic glucose sensor was integrated to the chip located at the back of the array. The sensor was assessed for glucose in MN-extracted simulated ISF from a reservoir in a petri dish, where the volume uptake was estimated gravimetrically as the mass loss in the petri dish. This sensor could determine glucose at a detection range between 0 and 35 mM at an accuracy within ±20% of the actual glucose concentration in sample, a sensitivity of 0.46 μA mM^{-1} and a limit of detection of 0.6 mM. In contrast to Mukerjee *et al.* and Zimmerman *et al.*, Strambini *et al.* showed that their device can perform rapid and quantitative analysis of glucose in ISF, although no in vivo evaluation was conducted. Nevertheless, drawbacks were seen in Strambini's system similar to those of Mukerjee *et al.*, including the need to move the sample outside the array for detection and micro-liter level of fluid, meaning a very small volume, making biomolecule analysis challenging.

Considering the drawbacks of the system designed by Mukerjee *et al.*, Ranamukhaarachchi *et al.* (2016) developed a point-of-care TDM device by integrating a gold-coated hollow microneedle with an optofluidic sensing system to detect vancomycin (a therapeutically monitored drug) in sub-nanoliter

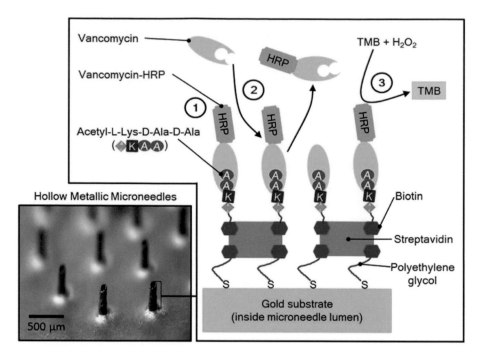

FIGURE 8.3 Functionalization of gold-coated hollow microneedle lumens for fluid collection, drug binding, and detection. (Figure obtained from Ranamukhaarachchi *et al.* (2016) with permission [22].)

volumes of fluid in vitro [22]. The coated needle's inner lumen was surface-functionalized with a vancomycin-specific peptide, which was then preloaded with a vancomycin-horseradish peroxidase (HRP) conjugate (Figure 8.3).

The functionalized microneedle device was integrated into the sensing elements, where a microfluidic chip consisting of a simultaneous detection chamber and an optical waveguide was equipped with micro-optical fibers for drug quantification using a simple absorbance scheme. During biological fluid collection, the sample filled the microneedle lumen volume of 0.6 nL by capillary action, which was significantly smaller than previously required sample volumes for sample analysis. Vancomycin present in the sample competed for the vancomycin-specific peptide on the lumen surface, and displaced the preloaded vancomycin-HRP conjugate. The remaining vancomycin-HRP was quantified by the 3,3′5,5′-tetramethylbenzidine (TMB) assay, where a TMB solution was passed through the lumen to cause a color change from clear to blue in the presence of vancomycin-HRP in a concentration-dependent manner. The magnitude of color change was determined by absorbance measurements in the optofluidic chamber requiring minute volumes (<50 nL) of TMB solution. Using this microneedle-optofluidic biosensor, Ranamukhaarachchi *et al.* demonstrated the potential of the sensor to assess vancomycin in its clinically relevant range (2.2–22.0 μM) with a high detection sensitivity (0.41 AU per 10 μM) and extremely low limit of detection of 84 nM. The signal-to-noise ratio of this system was extremely high, between 42.6 and 59.4 dB. The system's main advantages were the extremely low volume of fluid requirement, the capability to detect low-concentration TDM candidates with high signal-to-noise ratio, the rapid operation from collection to analysis (altogether less than 5 min TDM time), and the lack of need for sample transfer from the collection site to analysis. However, the system needs to be validated using preclinical and clinical studies.

8.3.3 Microneedle-Biosensors without Interstitial Fluid Extraction Requirements

Considering the challenges of extracting ISF, several research groups have developed MN-integrated biosensors for TDM and diagnostics purposes that did not require ISF extraction.

Corrie *et al.* (2010) developed a point-of-care diagnostic device to selectively extract biomarkers directly from the skin using solid microprojection arrays (MPAs), made by deep reactive ion etching of silicon, to eliminate the need for blood draws for diagnostics [5]. The device was evaluated on its capability to capture anti-Fluvax®-IgG antibody, 21 days after administration of the Fluvax® from the epithelia. Corrie *et al.* surface-functionalized the MPAs with thiolated PEG after coating the surface with a layer of gold, and grafted anti-Fluvax®-IgG capture proteins. After applying the MPAs for a period of 10 min in serum and in vivo in mouse ear skin, fluorescence intensity measurements on the MPA surfaces were determined by confocal microscopy. Further, the functionalized MPAs were assessed by an enzyme-linked immunosorbent assay (ELISA) method for anti-Fluvax®-IgG capture after insertion in mouse ear skin for 10 min. Sensitive detection capability of the anti-Fluvax®-IgG biomarker showed promise for the solid MN-based minimally invasive diagnostic devices. In addition, Muller *et al.* (2012) modified the surface of the MPAs to immobilize anti-NS1 monoclonal capture antibody to bind the NS1 antigen, which is a biomarker for dengue fever, in mice over a 20-min duration [23]. Using an ELISA assay in a 96-wellplate, the captured concentration of the NS1 biomarker was quantified at a detection limit of 8 µg mL^{-1}. Development of surface-functionalized MPAs has eliminated the need for a set volume of ISF collection for analysis, which is a significant advantage, given the limited availability of ISF in the skin. However, the prolonged duration for biomarker capture (10–20 min) and the need for expensive and large laboratory equipment, such as a confocal microscope and 96-wellplate readers for measurement, present drawbacks to using MPAs for diagnostics.

Windmiller *et al.* (2011) designed and developed an electrochemical biosensor using a two-component MN system, which included solid and hollow MN devices, for monitoring glutamate and glucose. Solid MNs were positioned inside the hollow MN, closing the lumen of the hollow MN and providing microcavities, where analyte-recognition enzymes (glutamate oxidase and glucose oxidase) were entrapped in a poly(*o*-phenylenediamine) film by an electropolymeric process [24]. This entrapment ensured the rejection of interfering electroactive compounds in the sample. The electrochemical sensor was assessed for detection of glutamate and glucose in vitro in a buffer solution and in undiluted human serum. The sensor measured the pathophysiological glutamate concentration range (0–140 µM) at a sensitivity of 8.1 nA µM^{-1} and a limit of detection of 21 µM. Similarly, the sensor detected glucose over its pathophysiological range from 0–14 mM at a sensitivity of 0.353 µA mM^{-1}, a limit of detection of 0.1 mM, and a signal-to-noise ratio of 3. Similarly to Keum *et al.* and Corrie *et al.*, the major benefit of this technology is the lack of need for extraction and sampling of biological fluids in monitoring and diagnostics applications.

Similarly, Miller *et al.* (2012) devised an all-in-one MN-based sensor for in vitro amperometric detection of pH, glucose, and lactate to monitor metabolic acidosis and presence of tumors [6]. Hollow MNs in an array were aligned with a well, which was filled with a carbon paste for sensing either pH, glucose, or lactate, and electrically isolated from one another. Change in pH, glucose concentration, and lactate concentrations in ISF-like physiological conditions (between pH 5 and 8) was detected by the carbon electrode in 0.1 M phosphate buffer against an external Ag/AgCl reference and Pt counter electrodes. However, the sensitivity of detection using this sensor (2.5 nA mM^{-1} glucose) was significantly lower than previously mentioned approaches. In addition, Miller *et al.* demonstrated the potential of a cell-resistant coating, called Lipidure®, to prevent biofouling of the sensors by macrophage adhesion, which is expected to increase the lifetime of the sensor in vivo when implanted as an array of sensing electrodes.

Keum *et al.* (2015) developed an MN sensor system (MSS) using a solid array connected to an endomicroscope for detection of colon cancer [4]. The MSS was fabricated using polycaprolactone, with coatings of polydopamine and poly(3,4-ethylenedioxythiophene), followed by functionalization of hemin molecules on the surface for nitric oxide (NO) binding and detection. Keum *et al.* confirmed the performance of the MSS for NO detection in vitro in simulated biological fluids and cell culture media, and in vivo in melanoma tissue. Further, when the MSS combined with the endomicroscope was inserted into mouse melanoma polyp regions, a sudden drop in the current detected by the electrical sensor was observed, in contrast to lack of significant current change in normal tissue. The MSS, operating at 100 mV, demonstrated detection of NO at a high sensitivity of 1.44 µA cm^{-2} µM^{-1} with a limit of detection of 1 µM NO to detect and distinguish cancer tissues in vivo from normal tissue in real time. Further developments to this MSS system for clinical applications will contribute significantly to improve early detection of cancers.

8.3.4 Continuous Monitoring Microneedle Devices

One of the most promising applications for MN-integrated biosensors is continuous monitoring of bio-molecules from the skin's ISF. Though some approaches described previously hinted at the possibility of continuous monitoring, this area of research and development remains to be explored in greater detail.

The first-ever MN-based continuous monitoring device that might be partially implanted in the epidermis was described by Jina *et al.* (2014), who developed a hollow MN-integrated continuous glucose monitoring (CGM) biosensor [25]. They demonstrated its capability accurately and continuously measured glucose concentrations in the body using ISF. The first prototype of the CGM biosensor consisted of a silicon MN array (~200 hollow projections), a glucose sensor, an electronics module, and a fluid flow system. The sensing chamber in Figure 8.4, which was located outside the cross-section of the skin, was filled with a proprietary buffer solution containing phosphate and citrate ions, to perform mutarotation of glucose and reduce the rate of wound healing in the skin due to the tissue damage caused by the MN insertion, respectively. In doing so, this CGM biosensor was designed to be inserted into the epidermal layer of skin to allow glucose present in the ISF to passively diffuse to an external glucose sensor located behind the array. This approach was unique among MN-integrated biosensors, since ISF extraction was not required as a primary function of the device.

The biosensor, currently being commercialized by Arkal Medical (Fremont, CA, USA), was clinically evaluated in 10 patients, who have received insulin treatment for over 16 years. CGM was done over periods of 48 h and 72 h, and measurements were compared with finger-stick blood glucose levels [25]. A lag of 17 min was found between the ISF glucose measurements and the blood glucose measurements, which was comparable to that of other commercialized subcutaneously implanted glucose

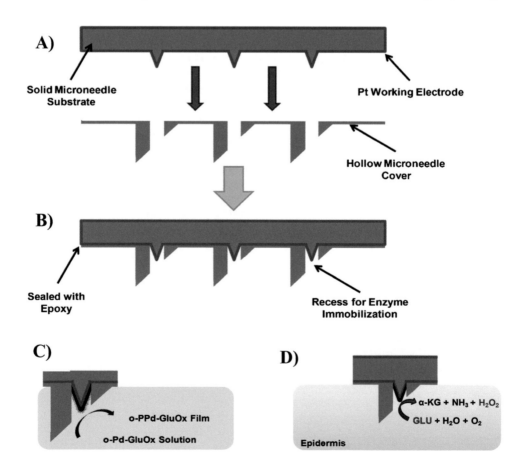

FIGURE 8.4 Continuous glucose-monitoring biosensor. (Figure obtained from Chua *et al.* (2013) with permission [26].)

sensors [27]. The method introduced and validated by Jina *et al.* for monitoring analytes in the ISF using hollow MNs can be applicable to and useful for other TDM candidate drugs to obtain real-time data to guide therapy.

8.4 Conclusions and Outlook

With predominant benefits of painless insertion, ability to extract ISF, presence of many biomolecules in ISF, and already identified correlations between ISF and blood for some biomolecules, microneedle-integrated biosensing devices have the potential to revolutionize diagnostics and TDM. Limited exploration of methodologies to utilize microneedles for minimally invasive biosensing has been performed to date, and though biosensing concepts have been presented previously with various MN technologies, the lack of preclinical and clinical validation on such systems presents gaps in knowledge on the performance of MN biosensors. It is envisioned that, similarly to the use of strategies employed in microneedle-based drug delivery systems, using unique microneedle strategies for biosensing will facilitate the development and commercialization of a plethora of novel devices for a multitude of applications. Combined with the movement toward digital health and wellness, it is likely that some MN technologies for continuous monitoring of biomolecules will be integrated to communicate with digital health trackers, such as mobile phones and activity watches. In contrast, other MN technologies will be used as single-use cartridges for point-of-care diagnostics. As the field of MN biosensors continues to grow over the next decade, more clinical and preclinical data, regulatory considerations, usability and human factors inputs, and biosensing applications will emerge to mark an exciting era for MN technologies.

REFERENCES

1. Touw, D., et al., *Cost-effectiveness of therapeutic drug monitoring: a systematic review.* Therapeutic Drug Monitoring, 2005. **27**(1): p. 10–17.
2. Kim, S.W., *Therapeutic drug monitoring (TDM) of antimicrobial agents.* Infection and Chemotherapy, 2008. **40**(3): p. 133–139.
3. Klonoff, D.C., *Continuous glucose monitoring roadmap for 21st century diabetes therapy.* Diabetes Care, 2005. **28**(5): p. 1231–1239.
4. Keum, D.H., et al., *Microneedle biosensor for real-time electrical detection of nitric oxide for in situ cancer diagnosis during endomicroscopy.* Advanced Healthcare Materials, 2015. **4**(8): p. 1153–1158.
5. Corrie, S.R., et al., *Surface-modified microprojection arrays for intradermal biomarker capture, with low non-specific protein binding.* Lab on a Chip, 2010. **10**(20): p. 2655–2658.
6. Miller, P.R., et al., *Multiplexed microneedle-based biosensor array for characterization of metabolic acidosis.* Talanta, 2012. 88: p. 739–742.
7. Marinova, M., et al., *Immunosuppressant therapeutic drug monitoring by LC-MS/MS: workflow optimization through automated processing of whole blood samples.* Clinical Biochemistry, 2013. 46(16): p. 1723–1727.
8. Seemann, S. and A. Reinhardt, *Blood sample collection from a peripheral catheter system compared with phlebotomy.* Journal of Infusion Nursing, 2000. **23**(5): p. 290–297.
9. Hallworth, M.W., I. Watson, *Therapeutic drug monitoring, Interactive clinical guide.* 3rd edition. Abbott Laboratories, Maidenhead, United Kingdom; 2017.
10. Kiang, T.K., U.O. Häfeli, and M.H. Ensom, *A comprehensive review on the pharmacokinetics of antibiotics in interstitial fluid spaces in humans: implications on dosing and clinical pharmacokinetic monitoring.* Clinical Pharmacokinetics, 2014. **53**(8): p. 695–730.
11. Kiang, T.K., et al., *Therapeutic drug monitoring in interstitial fluid: a feasibility study using a comprehensive panel of drugs.* Journal of Pharmaceutical Sciences, 2012. **101**(12): p. 4642–4652.
12. Jia, Y., et al., *Estimation of mycophenolic acid area under the curve with limited-sampling strategy in Chinese renal transplant recipients receiving enteric-coated mycophenolate sodium.* Therapeutic Drug Monitoring, 2017. **39**(1): p. 29.
13. Groenendaal, W., et al., *Quantifying the composition of human skin for glucose sensor development.* Journal of Diabetes Science and Technology, 2010. **4**(5): p. 1032–1040.

14. Wang, P.M., M. Cornwell, and M.R. Prausnitz, *Minimally invasive extraction of dermal interstitial fluid for glucose monitoring using microneedles.* Diabetes Technology and Therapeutics, 2005. **7**(1): p. 131–141.

15. Sakaguchi, K., et al., *A minimally invasive system for glucose area under the curve measurement using interstitial fluid extraction technology: evaluation of the accuracy and usefulness with oral glucose tolerance tests in subjects with and without diabetes.* Diabetes Technology & Therapeutics, 2012. **14**(6): p. 485–491.

16. Donnelly, R.F., et al., *Microneedle-mediated minimally invasive patient monitoring.* Therapeutic Drug Monitoring, 2014. **36**(1): p. 10–17.

17. Caffarel-Salvador, E., et al., *Hydrogel-forming microneedle arrays allow detection of drugs and glucose in vivo: potential for use in diagnosis and therapeutic drug monitoring.* PloS One, 2015. **10**(12): p. e0145644.

18. Romanyuk, A.V., et al., *Collection of analytes from microneedle patches.* Analytical Chemistry, 2014. **86**(21): p. 10520–10523.

19. Mukerjee, E., et al., *Microneedle array for transdermal biological fluid extraction and in situ analysis.* Sensors and Actuators A: Physical, 2004. **114**(2): p. 267–275.

20. Zimmermann, S., et al., *In-device enzyme immobilization: wafer-level fabrication of an integrated glucose sensor.* Sensors and Actuators B: Chemical, 2004. **99**(1): p. 163–173.

21. Strambini, L., et al., *Self-powered microneedle-based biosensors for pain-free high-accuracy measurement of glycaemia in interstitial fluid.* Biosensors and Bioelectronics, 2015. 66: p. 162–168.

22. Ranamukhaarachchi, S.A., et al., *Integrated hollow microneedle-optofluidic biosensor for therapeutic drug monitoring in sub-nanoliter volumes.* Scientific Reports, 2016. 6: p. 29075.

23. Muller, D.A., et al., *Surface modified microprojection arrays for the selective extraction of the dengue virus NS1 protein as a marker for disease.* Analytical Chemistry, 2012. **84**(7): p. 3262–3268.

24. Windmiller, J.R., et al., *Bicomponent microneedle array biosensor for minimally-invasive glutamate monitoring.* Electroanalysis, 2011. **23**(10): p. 2302–2309.

25. Jina, A., et al., *Design, development, and evaluation of a novel microneedle array-based continuous glucose monitor.* Journal of Diabetes Science and Technology, 2014. **8**(3): p. 483–487.

26. Chua, B., et al., *Effect of microneedles shape on skin penetration and minimally invasive continuous glucose monitoring in vivo.* Sensors and Actuators A: Physical, 2013. 203: p. 373–381.

27. Garg, S.K., M. Voelmle, and P.A. Gottlieb, *Time lag characterization of two continuous glucose monitoring systems.* Diabetes Research and Clinical Practice, 2010. **87**(3): p. 348–353.

9

Commercialized Microneedles

KangJu Lee
SeungHyun Park
Ji Yong Lee
Won Hyoung Ryu
School of Mechanical Engineering, Yonsei University

9.1 Factors Driving Microneedle (MN) Technology into the Market

Microneedle (MN) technology has been rigorously investigated during the last decade for various applications such as vaccination, cosmetics, pain treatments, ophthalmology, and many more. Recently, MN technology started rapidly moving from the research to commercial development stages. One of the reasons for such fast development is ascribed to the maturation of MN fabrication technology. The major portion of MN research in the beginning was focused on how to make MN structures using biocompatible polymers, metals, or ceramics. Now, after a decade of research, MN fabrication can be scaled up for mass production, and it can be even outsourced. Another factor can be found in the minimally invasive nature of MN-based drug delivery. The MNs penetrate through the epidermal and dermal layers, and they deliver drug into the tissue. In many cases, MNs are pulled out and they leave only drug beneath the dermal layer of the skin. This is a huge benefit for an FDA approval process compared to other drug-delivery methods whose devices remain in the human body. This expectation of shorter and possibly easier FDA approval processes makes MN technology attractive to many companies for commercial development. In addition, expandability of MN technology to a wide range of diseases is also a strong factor that drives the commercialization of MN technology for various diseases. Interestingly, since MN technology allows easy and relatively safe access to the inside of human body, it can also be used as a biomedical sensor to collect various biological information without expensive equipment or the aid of health care professionals. Thus, rapid commercialization efforts of MN technology in the biosensor field are also expected in the near future. In this chapter, various MN-related technologies will be introduced and their current efforts in commercialization development and clinical trials will be discussed.

9.2 Microneedle Injection System

Injection systems that use an MN to temporarily inject a drug formulation into the body are listed in Table 9.1. The MN injection system is based on an intradermal route by which a liquid or solid drug can be injected painlessly into the body using a hollow or solid MN with an applicator. As a one-time delivery system, it is different from a patch drug delivery system, which is attached to the skin and continuously releases drugs or injects drugs at regular intervals over a certain period. MN injection systems are divided into two types. First, a disposable injection unit with an applicator typically delivers a drug using a hollow MN that can be mounted on the applicator. Second, an integrated microinjection system, which is a combined system of the MN, prefilled reservoir, and applicator, delivers a drug into the body. In this chapter, the features, use, research, clinical trials, and certifications for the commercialization of MN injection systems are discussed.

TABLE 9.1

Microneedle Devices for Commercialization

	Manufacturer	Product	Certification	Drug and Purpose	Dimension	Remarks
Disposable injection unit with applicator	NanoPass Technologies Ltd.	MicronJet 600™	FDA 510(k) cleared, CE marked	Vaccine for polio, zoster, and influenza; insulin	MN height: 600 μm	Commercialized
	Debiotech	Debioject™	FDA phase 1 completed, CE marked	Pasteur® rabies vaccine	MN height: 350–900 μm; single MN or 3-MN array	
	NanoBioSciences	AdminPen™	unknown	Liquid formulations	MN height: 500–1400 μm; 31-to-187-MN array	Commercially available for clinical trials
	3M™	Hollow Microstructured Transdermal System (hMTS)	FDA phase 1 ongoing	Cancer vaccine (PAN-301-1)	MN height: 1500 μm; 12-MN array	Panacea Pharmaceuticals Inc. started FDA phase 1 clinical trials for intradermal injection of PAN-301-1: HAAH Nanoparticle Therapeutic Vaccine using 3M™ hMTS.
	Bayer HealthCare Pharmaceuticals Inc.	BETACONNECT™	FDA approved	BETASERON® (interferon beta-1b)	Needle diameter: 300 μm	Commercialized
Integrated microinjection system	Becton Dickinson	Soluvia™	FDA approved	Fluzone® (influenza vaccine)	MN height: 1500 μm	Sanofi Pasteur obtained FDA approval of Fluzone® Intradermal Quadrivalent Vaccine using BD Soluvia™. Commercialized
	Clearside Biomedical Inc.	SCS microinjector	FDA phase 3 completed	Triamcinolone acetonide (TA)	MN height: 700–800 μm	

(continued)

TABLE 9.1 (Continued)
Microneedle Devices for Commercialization

	Manufacturer	Product	Certification	Drug and Purpose	Dimension	Remarks
MN patch for cosmetics	Karatica Co., Ltd	I'm Fill Needle Patch	FDA human OTC drug	Hyaluronic acid, acetylhexapeptide-8 moisturizing, anti-aging	400-MN array	Commercialized
	Junmok International Co., Ltd.	Royal skin hyaluronic acid micro patch	FDA Human OTC drug	Hyaluronic acid, lactose moisturizing, anti-aging	MN height: 500–750 μm	Commercialized
	RAPHAS Co., Ltd	Acropass	FDA human OTC drug	Hyaluronic acid, EGF moisturizing, anti-aging	MN height: 350 μm; needle diameter: 30 μm	Commercialized
	Nissha Co., Ltd	Neo Basic HA Fill Micro Patch	–	Hyaluronic acid skin care	3600-MN array	Commercialized
MN patch for vaccination	Micron Biomedical, Inc	Micron Biomedical's microneedle patch	FDA phase 1 ongoing	Flu vaccination	MN height: 650 μm; base diameter: 200 μm; 100-MN array	
	Vaxxas	Nanopatch™	ANZCTR phase 1 ongoing	Vaccine, Fluvax®	20,000-MN array	
	Corium International, Inc.	MicroCor®	FDA phase 2a completed	PTH(1-34)	MN height: 200 μm	
	Zosano Pharma, Corp.	ADAM	FDA phase 3 ongoing	Zolmitriptan	MN height: 500 μm	
	Nemaura pharma, Ltd.	Micropatch™	Unknown	Vaccine	Unknown	
MN patch using micro-sized needle injection	Valeritas, Inc.	V-Go®	FDA 510(k) cleared	Insulin	Needle dimeter: 300 μm	Commercialized
	Nemaura Pharma, Ltd.	Memspatch Insulin Microneedle Device (IMD)	Unknown	Insulin	Unknown	
	SteadyMed, Ltd.	Trevyent™	Ready to resubmit for NDA approval	Treprostinil	Unknown	
	Enable Injections, Inc.	Enable Smart enFuse™	Unknwon	Various	Unknown	

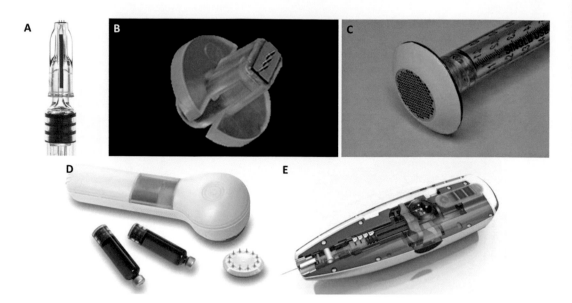

FIGURE 9.1 **(a)** MicronJet 600™ from NanoPass Technologies Ltd., **(b)** Debioject™ from Debiotech, **(c)** AdminPen™ from NanoBioSciences, **(d)** 3M™'s Hollow Microstructured Transdermal System (hMTS), and **(e)** BETACONNECT™ from Bayer HealthCare Pharmaceuticals Inc. Scale bar indicates 1 cm.

9.2.1 Disposable Injection Unit with an Applicator

A disposable injection unit with an applicator is a combination of a disposable MN and an applicator. As it is not a prefilled injection unit, any liquid formulation can be delivered. The injector of a disposable injection unit is divided into two concepts that are commercial syringes and customized applicators. In addition, a pen-type injection system has been developed, in which a commercial syringe is embedded in a pen-type injector, and the insertion depth or injection speed can be controlled.

As a painless intradermal injection system, a disposable unit connected to a syringe may be the first developed injection system that consists of a hollow MN unit and a standard commercial syringe. MicronJet 600™ from NanoPass Technologies Ltd. (Figure 9.1a), Debioject™ from Debiotech (Figure 9.1b), and AdminPen™ from NanoBiosciences (Figure 9.1c) are disposable MN units that can be mounted on the syringe tips. MicronJet 600™ is a pyramid-shaped hollow MN with a height of 600 μm for intradermal injections. Debioject™ is a microstructured hollow MN with a height of 350–900 μm that can infuse drug solutions into the dermis using a poke-and-flow approach. AdminPen™ is a planar MN with a height of 500–1400 μm and consists of a rectangular base and tapered tip. It is a solid MN and it creates a passage where the drug is delivered through the skin layer during the injection. For the lower cost of fabrication, these devices are manufactured by microfabrication technology. MicronJet 600™ is fabricated using a silicon etching technique to form a sharp tip [1]. Debioject™ was also developed using photolithography and deep silicon etching [2], and AdminPen™ uses electrochemical machining, electrical discharge machining, and other techniques [3]. MicronJet 600™ and Debioject™ are the most actively researched MNs. MicronJet 600™ has obtained FDA 510(k) clearance and CE mark, and Debioject™ is also a CE¹-marked MN device. MicronJet 600™ is currently undergoing FDA phase 2 clinical trials for allergy and cancer immunotherapy, and the varicella-zoster vaccine. MicronJet 600™ has demonstrated an improved immune response to an intramuscular full dose of Fluzone® with 4% to 40% of the intramuscular dose [4, 5]. Debioject™ completed FDA phase 1 clinical trial for intradermal rabies immunization using the vaccine Rabique Pasteur® with 20% of the standard intramuscular dose

---

¹ The CE mark indicates that the manufacturer of a product takes responsibility for the compliance of this product with all applicable European health, safety, performance and environmental requirements.

in 2015. A reduced dose of rabies vaccine administered with Debioject™ induced a humoral immune response similar to a full dose delivered by intramuscular injection with classical needles [2].

A disposable MN unit embedded in its customized applicator has been developed. The 3M™ hollow microstructured transdermal system (hMTS) (Figure 9.1d) and a multi-injection adaptor from Microdermics are disposable units which can be mounted in a customized applicator. 3M™'s polymeric hollow MN array is located on a 1.27-cm^2 circular base and consists of eighteen 500–900 μm microstructures [6]. Recently demonstrated models contain a polymer MN array with 12 hollow MNs, each approximately 1500 μm on 1 cm^2 of a circular base. The polymeric MN fabricated using a molding technique is mounted on a designed applicator consisting of a spring and liquid reservoir. The hMTS system delivers approximately 0.5–2 mL of pharmaceutical formulations, such as Cimzia®, Monoclonal AB, and protein, with an injection time of 1–5 min. Intradermal delivery using the hMTS had a larger immune response than that of intramuscular delivery [7]. The 3M™ human tolerability study showed that approximately 2 mL of the drug formulation could be delivered within 2 min using the hMTS [8]. In addition, Panacea Pharmaceuticals Inc. started FDA phase 1 clinical trial for intradermal injection of PAN-301-1: HAAH Nanoparticle Therapeutic Vaccine (cancer vaccine) using 3M™ hMTS in 2017. Microdermics has recently developed metallic hollow MNs using MEMS technology and fabricated a prototype of the disposable unit that can be connected to a commercial syringe. They demonstrated unique multi-injection adaptors and customized kits using their patented platform. In 2017, Microdermics entered a strategic agreement with contract development and manufacturing organization (CDMO), Vetter, for drug product manufacturing and packaging.

Finally, a pen-type injection system, in which an extremely long and slender needle is used, has been reported that can control the depth of insertion and the injection time, for example, the BETACONNECT™ electronic auto-injector from Bayer HealthCare (Figure 9.1e). BETACONNECT™ delivers BETASERON®, which is used to reduce relapsing-remitting multiple sclerosis (RRMS). A user can control the injection volume 0.25–1 mL of the drug at a depth of 8–12 mm using its FDA-approved smartphone application myBETAapp™ via Bluetooth technology. Bayer HealthCare conducted a study on patient satisfaction using BETACONNECT™. The user satisfaction score was higher than the conventional syringe injection for its ability to adjust the injection depth and speed [9]. In addition, as the first and only electronic auto-injector, Bayer HealthCare received FDA approval for BETACONNECT™ in 2015.

9.2.2 Integrated Microinjection Systems

An integrated microinjection system is a combined system of MNs and reservoirs that are prefilled with a desired drug, and syringes. Most integrated microinjection drug-delivery systems transfer liquid drug into the body (referred to as a prefillable microinjection system); however, solid MN injection using an applicator, referred to as separable MN injection, has also been demonstrated).

The first examples of an integrated microinjection system are the Soluvia™ from Becton Dickenson (BD) (Figure 9.2a) and the SCS (suprachoroidal space) microinjector from Clearside Biomedical Inc. (Figure 9.2b). The BD Soluvia™ prefillable microinjection system is a glass prefillable spring-based syringe system integrated with a 1.5 mm long 30 gauge stainless steel needle. The SCS microinjector is a prefillable suprachoroidal microinjection system with a height of approximately 700–800 μm for ocular injection. The SCS microinjector was fabricated from a 33G stainless steel needle with laser shaping and electropolishing [10]. BD conducted clinical trials involving more than 700 subjects and 3500 injections with BD Soluvia™ and demonstrated the safety and ease of use [11]. In addition, the BD clinical tests showed that the MN was barely perceptible when penetrating the skin, and effectively injected drug into the intradermal layer regardless of the subject's gender, ethnicity, and body mass [12]. Consequently, Sanofi Pasteur obtained FDA approval of Fluzone® Intradermal Quadrivalent (influenza vaccine) for adults using BD Soluvia™ in 2014. In addition, an FDA phase 3 clinical trial for suprachoroidal injection of CLS-TA (triamcinolone acetonide) in subjects with noninfectious uveitis (AZALEA) using the SCS microinjector has been completed in 2018.

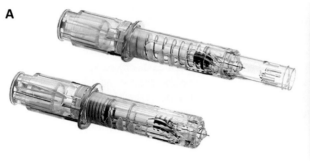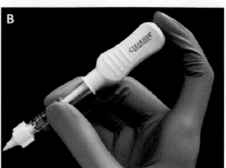

FIGURE 9.2   Soluvia™ from Becton Dickenson.

As another example, the JUVIC Microlancer device is a painless and patchless shooting microstructure that delivers solid insulin MNs directly into the body [13]. This spring-loaded system injects cone-shaped solid MNs into the tissue by detaching individual MNs from a thin substrate by punching MNs with pillars through the thin substrate. Injected MNs have a height of 600 μm and a bottom radius of 252 μm with an injection depth of approximately 50–100 μm in 50–100 ms. Microlancer overcomes the difficulties of complete injection through the thick hair-covered areas of the skin. A report on the progress of the clinical trials using Microlancer has not been published yet; however, it is an anticipated product that can achieve sustained drug delivery using a solid MN injection system.

9.3 Microneedle Patch System

9.3.1 Cosmetics

Recently, an MN patch has gained rapid momentum in the cosmetic field for skin moisturizing or anti-aging. Most of the commercialized MN patches are composed of HA that dissolves into the skin after administration. MNs made of HA can moisturize skin tissue and deliver small therapeutic molecules for skin improvement via their dissolution. Karatica Co., Ltd. developed an MN cosmetic patch for the treatment of tissue around the eyes and mouth. The I'm Fill Needle Patch contains over 400 HA needles with acetylhexapeptide-8 (Figure 9.3a). The Royal Skin Hyaluronic Acid Micro Patch developed by Junmok International Co., Ltd. is a HA MN patch that contains lactose and allows the ingredients to penetrate the stratum corneum (Figure 9.3b). The I'm Fill Needle Patch and Royal Skin Hyaluronic Acid Micro Patch obtained FDA Human OTC drug for moisturization and removal of fine wrinkles. RAPHAS Co., Ltd. has developed a HA-based dissolving microstructure patch, referred to as Acropass (Figure 9.3c). The backbone materials of the MN patch are the swellable polymer mixtures which contain epidermal growth factor for anti-aging. RAPHAS Co., Ltd. has international patents, including a droplet-born air blowing (DAB) method for fabrication of the Acropass MN [14]. The clinical trials showed positive outcomes in terms of the overall condition and elasticity improvement of skin after treatment by HA MN patches. The Acropass was also registered Human OTC drug in FDA. The Neo Basic HA Fill Micro Patch is based on the MicroCure®, dissolving MN technology of the Nissaha Co., Ltd. (Figure 9.3d). COSMETEX ROLAND Co., Ltd adopted the MicroCure® technology and developed MNs with flat-end shapes for greater safety.

9.3.2 Vaccination

An MN vaccine patch induces low pain, reduces administration times, and does not contain a cold-chain that might be affected by temperature variation during storage and transport. Micron

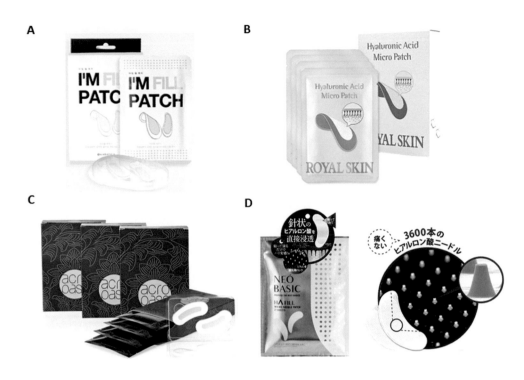

FIGURE 9.3 (a) Karatica Co., Ltd., I'm Fill Needle Patch, (b) Junmok International Co., Ltd., Royal Skin Hyaluronic Acid Micro Patch, (c) RAPHAS Co., Ltd., Acropass, (d) Nissha Co., Ltd., Neo Basic HA Fill Micro Patch.

Biomedical, Inc. and Vaxxas lead the development of vaccine-coated MN patches worldwide. Micron Biomedical's Microneedle Patch (Figure 9.4a), attached like a bandage, delivers dermal immune system cells into the skin to enhance the immune response in the epidermis. A phase 1 clinical trial for FDA approval showed that the Micron Biomedical's Microneedle Patch was safe and demonstrated an immune response as a flu vaccine. Vaxxas developed and commercialized Nanopatch™ for vaccine delivery that enables immune system activation below the skin surface (Figure 9.4b). Nanopatch™ consists of a 1 cm² square of silicon with approximately 20,000 vaccine-coated MNs on the surface. In a mouse model, the Nanopatch™ array increased immunogenicity with much reduced dose of Fluvax® (100-fold reduction was achieved) and higher vaccine efficacy was achieved. The Nanopatch™ is currently undergoing clinical trials for Australian New Zealand Clinical Trials Registry (ANZCTR).

Different types of MN applicators have been developed. Using an applicator, drug and vaccine could be delivered by a simple and one-step administration and the MN insertion pressure on the skin surface could be controlled. Corium International, Inc. has developed proprietary MicroCor® transdermal technology that utilizes dissolving MNs for drug delivery (Figure 9.4c). MicroCor® is fabricated by a combination of a water-insoluble backing layer and a solid-state biodegradable microstructure array containing an active therapeutic agent using the drug-in-tip technology. The MicroCor PTH(1-34) product, being developed for the treatment of osteoporosis, has successfully completed a phase 2a clinical evaluation. The Zosano Pharma Corp.'s patch system developed its unique microprojection array, called adhesive dermally applied microarray (ADAM) (Figure 9.4d). ADAM is mounted on the ZP-applicator and attached on the skin surface like an adhesive bandage. In the phase 1 clinical trial, ADAM showed a three-times-higher drug effect than that of the oral administration of Zolmitriptan for migraine treatment [15] and a phase 3 clinical trial has been conducted. Nemaura Pharma, Ltd. developed an advanced drug loading system, a solid dose delivery device called Micropatch™ (Figure 9.4e). Since the drugs are coated on the surface of the needle with a frustoconical-shaped pellet, Micropatch™ can deliver a solid dose below the skin. The

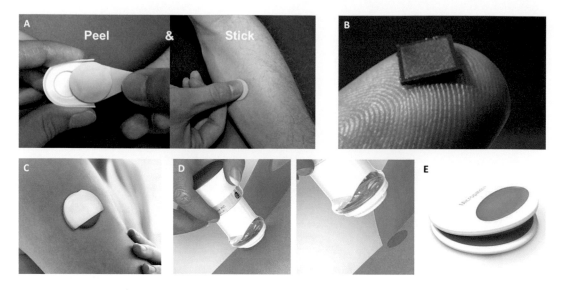

FIGURE 9.4 **(a)** Micron Biomedical, Inc., Micron Biomedical's Microneedle Patch, **(b)** Vaxxas, Nanopatch™, **(c)** Corium International, Inc., MicroCor®, **(d)** Zosano Pharma Corp., ADAM **(e)** Nemaura Pharma, Ltd., Micropatch™.

pellet is fabricated by compressing the combination of a freeze-dried vaccine and excipients using a micro-press to the desired size.

9.3.3 Micro-Sized Needle Injection Patch

For a patient who requires multiple and continuous drug delivery, patch-type needle injection devices that combined a micro-sized hypodermic needle have been developed. A patch-type applicator is able to sustain drug delivery while attached to the skin for dose control of drug delivery. Especially for a diabetic patient, a patch-type device decreases discomfort and amplifies drug efficacy owing to the automatic, continuous, and self-administered drug delivery. Valeritas, Inc. developed FDA 510(k) cleared V-Go®, a simple and disposable device for the delivery of basal-bolus insulin therapy (Figure 9.5a). V-Go® delivers insulin using 30-G hypodermic floating needle by pressing a button, without the use of batteries or complicated programming that help Type 2 diabetic patients easily control their glucose levels [16]. The Memspatch® insulin microneedle device (IMD) of Nemaura Pharma, Ltd. is an injector that infuses insulin by sliding the operating portion that reduces the patient's fear of needle pain (Figure 9.5b). Currently, the clinical trial showed that Memspatch® induced a lower pain level in Type 2 diabetic patients than other pen injectors.

SteadyMed, Ltd. has developed pump-type drug infusion devices utilizing hypodermic needles. The SteadyMed, Ltd.'s Trevyent™ is equipped with a self-powered expanding ECell® that pushes a piston and collapses the primary container that is filled with a sterile liquid drug (Figure 9.5c). SteadyMed, Ltd. was advised by the FDA to resubmit its new drug application (NDA) for Trevyent™ for the treatment of pulmonary arterial hypertension (PAH).

Finally, other micro-sized needle injection patches include Enable Injections, Inc.'s Enable Smart enFuse™ and Microdemics's Prefill Patch. Enable Smart enFuse™, which can store various volumes by selecting reservoir size, has a function that allows the user to pause the injection at any time (Figure 9.5d). Enable Smart enFuse™ is equipped with a reconstitution filling system that allows mixing/reconstitution and transferring of the lyophilized formulations or mixing of two liquid formulations. Microdermics also developed prototypes of needle patch devices called Prefilled Patch (Figure 9.5e), designed to enable pain-free injection and improvement of comfort and treatment to patients while attached on the skin. These devices contain various volumes of drugs and induce the dose-sparing effect of intradermal vaccine delivery.

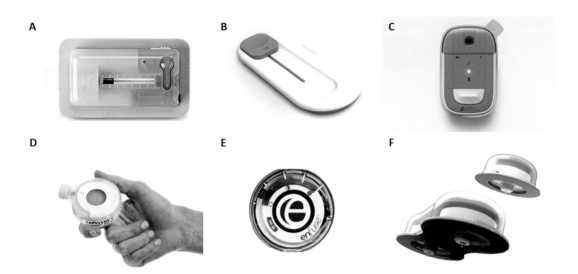

FIGURE 9.5 (a) Valeritas, Inc., V-Go®, (b) Nemaura Pharma, Ltd., Memspatch Insulin Microneedle Device (IMD), (c) SteadyMed, Ltd., Trevyent™, (d) Enable Injections, Inc., Enable Smart enFuse™, (e) Microdermics, Prefilled Patch.

9.4 Other Microneedle-Related Techniques

Several techniques have been developed and used over the past few decades for transdermal drug delivery enhancement, including sonophoresis, iontophoresis, and electroporation for improving the mode of drug delivery across the stratum corneum at the therapeutic level. However, these techniques have low efficiency of drug delivery. Since the first MNs were developed for transdermal use in 1998, they have been applied to the drug delivery field alone, and attempts have been made to improve transdermal drug delivery by combining the MNs with electrically driven technologies as well. Hollow or solid MNs can be pre-injected to provide a certain permeability increment, while a simultaneous ultrasound or electric field can enhance the flow rate via convection. Chen et al. attempted this combination (MNs with sonophoresis) to deliver calcein and BSA, and the enhancement showed drug permeability 9 times higher for calcein and 12 times higher for BSA than that of passive diffusion [17]. Han et al. used two sets of solid MNs to disrupt the skin surface and conducted sonophoresis. As a result, the permeability with the MN treatment was 2 times higher than that of a non-MN [18]. When an MN was integrated with iontophoresis, large molecular compounds were delivered to the skin or into the eye with high efficiency [19, 20]. Furthermore, in the field of electroporation, a commercialized product for a medical esthetic application, an electroporation needle (EPN) was developed by Eunsung Global Corporation (Figure 9.6a). An EPN has an MN array (9 MNs and a 200-µm diameter) at the end of an electroporation applicator. The array is repeatedly injected at a rate of 4000–6000 times per minute, and the penetration depth can be adjusted from 100 to 2000 µm, with respect to the target tissue. Because of the fractioned microneedling treatment combined with the electroporation treatment, the EPN improves the delivery of the active substances in the different layers of the facial skin and scalp.

MNs have also been developed for the delivery of drugs to vascular tissues. Arteries and veins have three layers: the adventitia (the outermost layer), the tunica media (the middle layer), and the endothelium (the innermost layer). The main factor that induces vascular disease is the narrowing of the blood vessels caused by abnormal growth of the smooth muscle cells (SMCs) that exist within the tunica media. Therefore, treatment to prevent the proliferation of SMCs requires the delivery of anti-proliferative drugs to the middle layer. Direct vascular drug delivery routes are either perivascular (via the outermost layer) or endovascular (via the innermost layer). Both methods have drawbacks owing to the micron-scale thickness of the adventitia and endothelium,

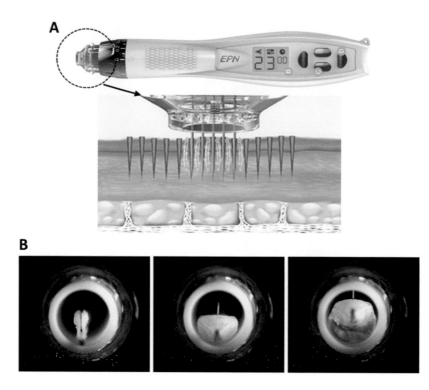

FIGURE 9.6 **(a)** Electroporation microneedle (EPN) system, Eunsung Global Corporation and **(b)** Bullfrog® micro-infusion device, Mercator.

which act as physical barriers. A novel MN [21] cuff and MN mesh [22] have been studied to enhance the efficiency of drug delivery compared to that of conventional perivascular-wrap-type devices. A drug-coated MN array attached to a curved poly(lactic-co-glycolic) acid (PLGA) film can achieve conformal contact with the vascular tissue and increase the efficiency of drug delivery 200 times higher than that of a flat film device (non-MN). A flexible mesh device with an MN array enhances the wrappable mountability surrounding the perivascular region with the strength of MN drug delivery. In endovascular drug delivery, the Mercator Bullfrog® micro-infusion device was introduced by combining a 34G micro-scale needle with a balloon catheter (Figure 9.6b). The Bullfrog device is tipped with a balloon-sheathed MN. When the desired injection site is reached, the balloon is inflated to 2 atm, securing the system for injection and sliding the MN through the vessel wall. The Bullfrog device has received 510(k) clearance from the FDA and CE mark in 2016.

In addition to the drug delivery field, biosensing of target analytes in interstitial fluid (ISF) is an emerging field for MN applications. ISF has been extensively explored for metabolites, such as glucose and lactate [23, 24]. Continuous glucose monitoring (CGM) has been extensively studied, and there is good clinical evidence that effective CGM in Type 1 diabetic patients leads to a reduced frequency of hypoglycemic episodes and lowered HbA1c [25]. Intensive treatment of diabetes reduces the risk of complications [26, 27], and glucose monitoring is a core component of successful management, especially for those who are insulin-dependent. Despite the promise of minimally invasive continuous monitoring, the CGM use of some of the approved commercial devices, such as those from Medtronic (Enlite), Dexcom (G5), and Abbott (FreeStyle Libre), is < 10% [28, 29]. This can be attributed to poor accuracy and precision (numerous false alarms) and high manufacturing costs. An MN patch platform allows the device to be in constant contact with the skin, providing permanent access to the ISF and enabling the device to operate continuously [30]. The short length of the MNs creates optimal penetration for ISF sensing, as the

MNs do not reach the dermis layer. This minimizes damage to the blood capillaries and nerve endings found in the dermis layer. Moreover, as the MNs penetrate the skin, sweat contamination is avoided [30]. Although this study remains in a research stage, the tests have shown that this device can operate successfully for up to 72 h with a 17-min lag time caused by the passive diffusion of the analytes from the blood into the ISF matrix [31]. To increase the lifetime of the device, the skin healing process must be inhibited. This might be achieved by designing a sensing patch with MNs of optimal length, width, tip, and pitch characteristics and by coating the MNs with a biocompatible material exhibiting mechanical properties similar to that of biological tissue. Currently, the device must be recalibrated daily using the finger-prick method [31]. Potential clogging of the MNs and the distortion of their shape upon penetration of the skin can also affect the dynamics of sampling. Despite these drawbacks, this novel device has great potential for a noninvasive CGM.

9.5 Commercial and Clinical Development of Microneedles

As summarized in Table 9.1, there are a number of commercialized MN products available in the market. MN injection systems such as MicronJet 600™, Debioject™, BETACONNECT, and Soluvia™ are FDA-cleared and now available as products. Cosmetic MN patches are also in the market such as the I'm Fill Patch from Karatica Co., Ltd. and Royal Skin Hyaluronic Acid Micro Patch from Junmok International Co., Ltd. for moisturizing and anti-aging. The V-Go from Valeritas Inc., an insulin delivery needle system, is also on sale for diabetes treatment. On the other hand, most of the MN techniques described thus far have completed phase 1 clinical trials and are performing the next-level clinical trials. To explore the trends of the recent MN development for clinical applications, this section examines the MN technology at the initial development stages: phase 1 or N/A. "N/A" is used to describe trials without FDA-defined phases, including trials of devices or behavioral interventions. From the database of the U.S. National Library of Medicine and International Clinical Trials Registry Platform, ongoing or before-phase-1 data of clinical trials related to the MN were investigated and analyzed. The screened MN developments can be classified into five categories according to similar technologies: the MN patch, the radio frequency (RF) MN, microneedling, the suprachoroidal space (SCS) injection MN, and MN injection into the gingiva (Table 9.2).

The research spectrum using an MN patch is broad, including the comparison of vaccinations with a hypodermic needle, various drug delivery trials, the effect of the MN patch injection, and finally the MN for continuous glucose monitoring. An inactivated influenza vaccine was injected into a healthy adult for a comparative study with a hypodermic vaccine (NCT02438423). In another study, in situ MN array-directed chemo-immunotherapy using doxorubicin was conducted to eliminate tumor cells (NCT02192021). In addition, various immunotherapies (NCT02837094) and stem cells (NCT02329457) have been delivered using an MN patch. As MN patch drug delivery has increased, further research has been conducted. The insertion mechanism of an MN patch with respect to the ethnicity was examined to define the rate of skin barrier recovery following an MN treatment (NCT03332628). Integrated with a topical ointment treatment, the study of therapeutic efficacy using a hyaluronic acid MN patch was conducted to enhance the efficacy of the patch on the psoriatic plaques (NCT02955576). In addition to transdermal drug delivery, the MN patch has been applied in the biosensing field. A comparative study with three glucose measurement techniques, including an intravenous catheter, lancet, and MN patch, was registered in the NIH. This study aimed to determine if an MN patch, as against a lancet or intravenous catheter, would be a preferable option for monitoring glucose levels for the diabetic pediatric population (NCT02682056).

The MN integrating electrostimulation RF is an emerging technology for the clinical market. The main target application of this technique is cosmetic, such as the reduction of wrinkles or striae alba or the treatment of acne. Male and female patients with neck wrinkle indications from 25 to 65 years of age were evaluated (ChiCTR-INR-16010169). The patient or guardian voluntarily signed the informed

TABLE 9.2

Microneedles in Early Clinical Trials

Related Technology	Main ID	Primary Sponsor	Phase	Study Title	Intervention/ Treatment	Brief Summary and Primary Outcome (bold)
MN patch	NCT02668056	Emory University	N/A	Glucose Measurement Using Microneedle Patches	Device: Intravenous (IV) catheter Device: Lancet Device: Microneedle patch	• Comparison of three glucose measurement techniques • To determine whether an MN patch (made from biocompatible polymers or metal) would be preferable to a lancet or intravenous catheter **Superior glucose level of MN patch**
	NCT02955576	The Catholic University of Korea	N/A	Efficacy of Microneedle Patch on Topical Ointment Treatment of Psoriasis	Device: Microneedle HA patch Device: Patch	• To evaluate the efficacy of MN patch on the psoriatic plaques **Improvement of psoriasis**
	NCT03332628	University of Iowa	N/A	Racial/Ethnic Differences in Microneedle Response	Device: Microneedle HA patch	• To define the rate of skin barrier recovery following MN treatment of the skin in healthy subjects of differing racial/ ethnic backgrounds **Micropore closure kinetics**
	NCT02438423	Mark Prausnitz	1	Inactivated Influenza Vaccine Delivered by Microneedle Patch or by Hypodermic Needle	Biological: Inactivated influenza vaccine using MN patch	• Inactivated influenza vaccination (IIV) with MN patch and hypodermic needle) or placebo (by MN patch) • Investigation of safety, reactogenicity, acceptability, and immunogenicity **To evaluate the safety and reactogenicity following receipt of inactivated influenza vaccine delivered by MN patch (either by staff or self-administered)**
	NCT02192021	Falo, Louis, MD	1	Micro Needle Array-Doxorubicin (MNA-D) in Patients with Cutaneous T-Cell Lymphoma (CTCL) (MNA-D)	Device: Microneedle array— Doxorubicin (MNA-D)	• In situ MNA-directed chemo-immunotherapy using doxorubicin for termination of tumor cells locally **Safety of the MNA-D system** **Measurement of vital signs, hematology, comprehensive metabolic panel, assessment for skin toxicity, and adverse event evaluation**
	NCT02837094	Cardiff University	1	Enhanced Epidermal Antigen Specific Immunotherapy Trial-1 (EE-ASI-1)	Drug: C19-A3 GNP	• C19-A3 GNP peptide administration via Nanopass MNs **To examine the risk of C19A3 GNP administration in terms of general safety and induction of hypersensitivity**
	NCT02329457	The University of Hong Kong	N/A	VZV Vaccine for Hematopoietic Stem Cell Transplantation (VZIDST)	Biological: Zostavax	• Direct vaccination of hematopoietic stem cell transplantation • Assessment of the efficacy and safety of the novel intradermal live-attenuated VZV vaccination using MN patch **Immunological response in donors**

TABLE 9.2 (Continued)
Microneedles in Early Clinical Trials

Related Technology	Main ID	Primary Sponsor	Phase	Study Title	Intervention/ Treatment	Brief Summary and Primary Outcome (bold)
Radio frequency (RF) MN	ChiCTR-INR-16010169	Shanghai Ninth People's Hospital, Shanghai Jiaotong University School of Medicine	N/A	The Treatment of Neck Wrinkles with Microneedle Radiofrequency Device: A Prospective, Randomized, Self-Controlled Clinical Trial	Device: RF MN	• To reduce neck wrinkles from the patient, 25–65 years old, both male and female • Exclusion of those who are pregnant or have anesthetic allergy or skin ulceration **Evaluation scale for aged skin of the neck**
	IRCT2014101519543N1	Vice Chancellor for Research, Isfahan University of Medical Sciences	N/A	Treatment of Stria Alba by Micro Needle Radio-Frequency Device	Device: RF MN	• Comparison of RF MN plus fractional CO$_2$ laser efficacy versus RF MN device alone in treatment of stria alba **Stria alba lesions**
	NCT03426098	Goldman, Butterwick, Fitzpatrick and Groff	N/A	Secret Micro-Needle Fractional RF System® for the Treatment of Facial Wrinkles	Device: Secret Micro-Needle Fractional RF System®	• To assess the safety, efficacy, and patient satisfaction associated with the treatment of facial wrinkles using RF MN (Ilooda Co., Ltd., Suwon, South Korea) **Improvement in Wrinkles Based on the Fitzpatrick Wrinkle Scale**
	NCT03380845	Massachusetts General Hospital	N/A	Comparison of 1550-nm Laser and Fractional Radiofrequency Microneedle for the Treatment of Acne Scars in Ethnic Skin	Device: Fraxel Restore Device: Fractora	• To compare the efficacy and safety of a erbium-doped 1550 nm non-ablative fractional laser and a bipolar fractional RF MN device for the treatment of atrophic facial acne scars in ethnic skin (Fitzpatrick Skin Phototypes III-VI) **Improvement in acne scarring**

(continued)

TABLE 9.2 (Continued)
Microneedles in Early Clinical Trials

Related Technology	Main ID	Primary Sponsor	Phase	Study Title	Intervention/ Treatment	Brief Summary and Primary Outcome (bold)
Micro-needling	NCT02660320	Centre Hospitalier Universitaire de Nice	N/A	Comparison of the Efficacy of Micro-Holes vs. Laser-Assisted Dermabrasion, for Repigmenting in Vitiligo Skin Dermabrasion	Device: Dermabrasion	• To compare the efficacy of laser-assisted dermabrasion + autologous epidermal cells suspension grafting versus dermabrasion using microneedling technique + autologous epidermal cells suspension grafting **Rate of repigmentation lesions**
	NCT03390439	Hospital de Clinicas de Porto Alegre	N/A	Treatment of Atrofic Striae with Percutaneous Collagen Induction Therapy versus Fractional Nonablative Laser	Device: Nd:YAP 1340 nm laser Device: Microneedling	• To evaluate the response of MN and fractional non-ablative laser Nd:YAP 1340 nm in the treatment of abdominal striae alba **Clinical response in abdominal alba striae after the therapies**
	NCT02962180	Mohammed V Souissi University	N/A	Transplantation of Basal Cell Layer Suspension Using Derma-Rolling System in Vitiligo	Device: Dermabrasion with dermaroller	• To develop a novel method for transepidermally delivering keratinocytes and melanocytes into vitiligo skin using derma-rolling system. **Rate of repigmentation lesions**
	NCT03409965	Lutronic Corporation	N/A	Lutronic Infini and LaseMD Systems in Combination Treatment	Device: Dermabrasion with dermaroller	• To evaluate the safety and effectiveness of the Infini and LaseMD Systems for combination treatment in wrinkles, texture, and pigmentation of the face and/or neck **Masked, qualitative assessment of improvement**
SCS injection MN	NCT02952001	Clearside Biomedical, Inc.	N/A	Extension Study of Patients with Non-infectious Uveitis Who Participated in CLS1001-301	Disease Models	• To characterize the continued clinical benefit regarding safety and efficacy of suprachoroidally administered CLS-TA, triamcinolone acetonide A non-interventional extension study of up to 6 months for subjects completing the parent study **Time to additional therapy for uveitis**
MN injection	NCT03274674	Bezmialem Vakif University	N/A	Use of Injectable-Platelet-Rich-Fibrin (I-PRF) to Thicken Gingival Phenotype	Other: I-PRF	• To investigate whether for individuals with thin gingival thickness who are susceptible to gingival recession, the use of I-PRF with MN increases gingival thickness without the need for surgical procedures **Gingival thickness**

consent and performed a self-controlled experiment with a follow-up using RF MNs. In the past few years, fractional RF systems have been introduced to enable controlled skin resurfacing accompanied with dermal collagen remodeling. Facial wrinkles were treated using the Secret Micro-Needle Fractional RF System® from Cryomed (NCT03426098). Striae alba reduction was performed using MN RF plus a fractional CO_2 laser (IRCT2014101519543N1). A fractional RF MN for the treatment of acne scars on ethnic skin was studied at Massachusetts General Hospital and was compared with conventional laser treatment devices (NCT03380845).

Even though advanced technologies have been developed, such as dermabrasion using a laser, microneedling has become the essential procedure of the pretreatment of the skin for various purposes. Many studies have shown promising results for the treatment of acne scars with a nonablative fractional laser and microneedling. A comparative study has been conducted with a fractional Nd:YAP 1340 nm laser and microneedling for the treatment of abdominal striae alba (NCT03390439). An evaluation of the microholes from microneedling has been performed by a comparison of laser-assisted dermabrasion for treating repigmentation of the skin (NCT02660320). In addition to these comparative experiments with existing technologies, microneedling enhances the efficiency of drug delivery in combination with laser technologies. For derma-rolling, tiny micro-injuries in the epidermis could offer a minimally invasive and painless method of cell transplantation (NCT02962180). A combination of laser dermabrasion and microneedling is under clinical evaluation as well (NCT03409965).

The SCS MN injection was developed and clinically demonstrated by Clearside Biomedical. They have performed several clinical trials for the commercialization of an MN injector for drug delivery through SCS. Recently, a clinical study was conducted to characterize the continued clinical benefit regarding the safety and efficacy of suprachoroidally administered CLS-TA, a triamcinolone acetonide injectable suspension, for the treatment of macular edema associated with noninfectious uveitis (NCT02952001). The parent study is a phase 3 multicenter study to assess the safety and efficacy of 4 mg of CLS-TA administered via suprachoroidal injection. Drug delivery to new sites using an MN injection platform rather than a percutaneous method has also been clinically evaluated. Injectable platelet-rich fibrin (I-PRF) has been administrated using an MN injector in the gingiva of patients susceptible to gingival recession (NCT03274674).

9.6 Conclusions

In this chapter, the current states of MN products and technologies for commercial development were surveyed. There are a number of commercialized MN products including MN injection systems, cosmetic MN patches, and MN insulin delivery systems. Combinatory products such as MN with RF-based technology and MN-integrated balloon catheter for endovascular drug delivery were also introduced to the market. MN systems for various therapeutic purposes other than vaccination or cosmetics are in either preclinical or clinical trials and FDA clearance is expected soon. These include RF MN or microneedling for cosmetics, SCS injection MN for ocular drug delivery, and MN for dental drug delivery. Microneedle-based biosensing such as minimally invasive CGM for diabetes treatment is another potential market.

REFERENCES

1. Levin, Yotam, et al. "Intradermal vaccination using the novel microneedle device MicronJet600: past, present, and future." Human vaccines & immunotherapeutics 11.4 (2015): 991–997.
2. Vescovo, Paul, et al. "Safety, tolerability and efficacy of intradermal rabies immunization with DebioJect™." Vaccine 35.14 (2017): 1782–1788.
3. Yuzhakov, Vadim V. "Method of making microneedle array and device for applying microneedle array to skin." U.S. Patent No. 8,414,548. 9 Apr. 2013.

4. Hung, Ivan FN, et al. "Dose sparing intradermal trivalent influenza (2010/2011) vaccination overcomes reduced immunogenicity of the 2009 H1N1 strain." Vaccine 30.45 (2012): 6427–6435.

5. Beals, Chan R., et al. "Immune response and reactogenicity of intradermal administration versus subcutaneous administration of varicella-zoster virus vaccine: an exploratory, randomised, partly blinded trial." The lancet infectious diseases 16.8 (2016): 915–922.

6. Burton, Scott A., et al. "Rapid intradermal delivery of liquid formulations using a hollow microstructured array." Pharmaceutical research 28.1 (2011): 31–40.

7. Fuller, Steven, et al. "Enhanced immunogenicity of a nanoparticle therapeutic cancer vaccine targeting HAAH delivered intradermally using 3M's hollow microstructured transdermal system (hMTS)." Journal for immunotherapy of cancer 3.2 (2015): P433.

8. Dick, Lisa A. et al. "Innovative drug delivery technology to meet evolving need of biologics & small moledules." *ONdrugDelivery* 56 (2015): 4–7.

9. Ziemssen, Tjalf, et al. "Patient satisfaction with the new interferon beta-1b autoinjector (BETACONNECT™)." Neurology and therapy 4.2 (2015): 125–136.

10. Kim, Yoo C. et al. "Targeted delivery of antiglaucoma drugs to the supraciliary space using microneedles." Investigative ophthalmology & visual science 55.11 (2014): 7387–7397.

11. Laurent, Philippe E., et al. "Evaluation of the clinical performance of a new intradermal vaccine administration technique and associated delivery system." Vaccine 25.52 (2007): 8833–8842.

12. Laurent, Aurélie, et al. "Echographic measurement of skin thickness in adults by high frequency ultrasound to assess the appropriate microneedle length for intradermal delivery of vaccines." Vaccine 25.34 (2007): 6423–6430.

13. Jung, Hyung Il, et al. "Painless and patchless shooting microstructure." U.S. Patent Application No. 15/028,007.

14. Kim, Jung Dong, et al. "Droplet-born air blowing: novel dissolving microneedle fabrication." Journal of controlled release 170.3 (2013): 430–436.

15. Kellerman, Donald J., Mahmoud Ameri, and Stewart J. Tepper. "Rapid systemic delivery of zolmitriptan using an adhesive dermally applied microarray." Pain management 7.6 (2017): 559–567.

16. Kapitza, Christoph, et al. "Basal—prandial insulin delivery in type 2 diabetes mellitus via the V-Go™: a novel continuous subcutaneous infusion device." Journal of diabetes science and technology 2.1 (2008): 40–46.

17. Chen, Bangtao, et al. "Sonophoretic enhanced microneedles array (SEMA)—Improving the efficiency of transdermal drug delivery." Sensors and Actuators B: Chemical 145.1 (2010): 54–60.

18. Han, Tao, et al. "Permeability enhancement for transdermal delivery of large molecule using low-frequency sonophoresis combined with microneedles." Journal of pharmaceutical sciences 102.10 (2013): 3614–3622.

19. Todo, Hiroaki, et al. "The synergistic effect of iontophoresis or electroporation and microneedles on the skin permeation of high molecular weight compounds." Percutaneous Penetration Enhancers Physical Methods in Penetration Enhancement. Springer, Berlin, Heidelberg, 2017. 379–387.

20. Jung, J. H. et al. "Iontophoretic targeting of drug delivery in the eye via the suprachoroidal space." Acta ophthalmologica 95.S259 (2017).

21. Lee, Kang Ju, et al. "Perivascular biodegradable microneedle cuff for reduction of neointima formation after vascular injury." Journal of controlled release 192 (2014): 174–181.

22. Lee, JiYong, et al. "Transfer-molded wrappable microneedle meshes for perivascular drug delivery." Journal of controlled release 268 (2017): 237–246.

23. Ciechanowska, Anna, et al. "Microdialysis monitoring of glucose, lactate, glycerol, and pyruvate in patients with diabetic ketoacidosis." The international journal of artificial organs 36.12 (2013): 869–877.

24. Miller, Philip R., et al. "Hollow microneedle-based sensor for multiplexed transdermal electrochemical sensing." Journal of visualized experiments: JoVE 64 (2012): e4067.

25. Pickup, John C, et al. "Glycaemic control in type 1 diabetes during real time continuous glucose monitoring compared with self monitoring of blood glucose: meta-analysis of randomised controlled trials using individual patient data." BMJ 343 (2011): d3805.

26. Diabetes Control and Complications Trial Research Group. "The effect of intensive treatment of diabetes on the development and progression of long-term complications in insulin-dependent diabetes mellitus." New England journal of medicine 329.14 (1993): 977–986.

27. UK Prospective Diabetes Study (UKPDS) Group. "Intensive blood-glucose control with sulphonylureas or insulin compared with conventional treatment and risk of complications in patients with type 2 diabetes (UKPDS 33)." The lancet 352.9131 (1998): 837–853.

28. Heinemann, Lutz, et al. "Reimbursement for continuous glucose monitoring: a European view." Journal of diabetes science and technology 6.6 (2012): 1498–1502.

29. Lodwig, Volker, et al. "Current trends in continuous glucose monitoring." Journal of diabetes science and technology 8.2 (2014): 390–396.

30. Coyle, Shirley, et al. "Wearable bio and chemical sensors." Wearable sensors (2015): 65–83.

31. Jina, Arvind, et al. "Design, development, and evaluation of a novel microneedle array-based continuous glucose monitor." Journal of diabetes science and technology 8.3 (2014): 483–487.

10

Considerations for Clinical Trials Involving Microneedle Devices

Janet Tamada
Scientia Bioengineering Consulting

10.1 Introduction

Microneedle technology has made significant progress for cosmetic enhancement of skin appearance, painless delivery of drugs and vaccines (1, 2), and accessing the myriad of analytes in skin interstitial fluid for physiological monitoring or diagnosis (3). Human clinical testing is an essential part of developing microneedle products. This chapter focuses on considerations for human clinical trials involving microneedles, including system design, manufacturing, biological interface, and ethical and regulatory requirements for clinical testing.

Prausnitz (4) proposed a useful framework of different modes of microneedle use that incorporates the microneedle design and the transport mechanism of the active agent (drug or vaccine) or analyte. This is adapted below:

- Solid microneedle arrays for pretreatment ("poke and place") are applied to disrupt the skin barrier, and a drug-containing or -sensing patch is placed over the disrupted skin.
- Coated, dissolving, or degrading microneedle arrays ("poke and remove") are applied to the skin, the needle coating or microneedle array dissolves to deliver the active agent, and the depleted array is removed.
- Hollow microneedles ("poke and push") are applied and active agent in a fluid is pushed through the bores of the needles.
- Microneedles with conduits, such as a hydrogel that allows diffusion or a hollow microneedle, are left in the skin for extended duration ("poke and leave"), allowing continuous analyte sensing or delivery of active agents.

For drugs and vaccines, clinical development typically involves three phases (5). Phase I testing evaluates safety and pharmacokinetics or immune response of the drug or vaccine, respectively, delivered by the microneedle route of administration in a small number of healthy volunteers. Phase II testing is performed on a larger group of patients in the target population and determines the dose range for efficacy of the drug or immune response to the vaccine. Phase III testing establishes the safety and efficacy of the final formulation and product design in a larger patient population. For medical devices, clinical development typically involves early-stage feasibility or pilot studies, which are performed on a small subject population using prototypes of the device, and late-stage pivotal studies with the final device design, which are performed on a larger subject pool of the target population.

10.2 Design Considerations

10.2.1 Penetration of Microneedles into the Skin

Microneedles must penetrate the outer layer of skin in order to be effective, and must remain intact so they do not leave fragments in the skin. The skin is elastic and deforms around the needles, making reliable penetration challenging. Two main approaches have been used to apply needles to ensure penetration (6):

- Using sufficiently long (> 600 μm), sharp microneedles so that low force is required to penetrate the skin and application can be achieved manually.
- Using a high-impact application device to drive the needles through the skin at high velocity.

Techniques such as dye staining, transepidermal water loss (TEWL) measurements, skin conductance measurements, and optical coherence tomography (OCT) have been used to evaluate penetration success (7).

10.2.2 After Microneedles Penetrate the Skin: Mode of Use

The mode of microneedle use drives many design activities. If the microneedles are removed and a patch system is applied ("poke and place"), then a positioning mechanism, such as marker or appliance, that enables the user to place the patch over the pretreated area must be developed and active agent or analyte transport rate over time must be measured to determine how long the system maintains active. For coated or dissolving microneedles ("poke and remove"), the limited capacity of a few milligrams restricts their use to potent active agents. A formulation must be developed to ensure that the dissolution time and the amount of residual active agent on used arrays or deposited on the skin surface are acceptable for the intended use. For hollow microneedle systems with fluid injection ("poke and push"), injection pressure and fluid volume limitations must be considered. Hollow microneedles can readily inject fluid volumes of up to a few hundred microliters, but volumes of 1 mL encounter resistance as the skin deforms to accommodate the fluid volume (8, 9) and two mL has required an infusion system (10). For microneedle arrays that are left in the skin ("poke and leave"), wear duration is limited to about one week due to shedding of the outer layer of skin, perspiration, and movement, which dislodge the needles. *In vitro* and animal models of adhesion to human skin have had limited predictive capabilities, so human clinical testing is required to determine adhesive wear properties of the system.

10.2.3 Design for Usability: Human Factors and Patient Acceptance

Microneedles have shown good patient acceptability, as they do not penetrate to a depth to activate the pain receptors in the skin (7). This creates an opportunity to design products that require minimal training, such as for self-administration or for regions with limited access to trained medical personnel. Late-phase clinical and summative human factors studies are employed to validate that the intended population can use the product with the supplied training materials (11–13). For example, testing may evaluate ability of users to perform the application steps correctly, keep the system on the skin long enough for the active agent to be delivered, or dispose of the used needles properly.

10.3 Manufacturing Process Considerations

10.3.1 General Manufacturing Controls

Manufacturers must use good manufacturing practices that are appropriate for the phase of development to ensure the safety, potency, and purity of the drug or vaccine (14, 15) or safety and functionality of a device clinical product (16). Microneedle products delivering active agent are considered drug–device combination products and must conform to requirements of both drugs or biologics and medical devices (17). Content uniformity of 85% to 115% of target dose (18) can be particularly challenging for processing the minute doses involved in microneedle products (19).

10.3.2 Bioburden Control

As microneedles pose a risk of infection, a low bioburden or sterility (20) and appropriate packaging (21, 22) will be required for regulatory approval. This affects the formulation, design, and processing of microneedle products. Some products can undergo terminal sterilization, such as steam, dry heat, electron beam or gamma irradiation, or ethylene oxide exposure, in which the product is sterilized after it has been manufactured and packaged (23). However, some analyte-sensing chemistries, many drugs, and most biologics do not retain their activity after sterilization, and require aseptic processing (24). Aseptic processing involves manufacturing in highly controlled, clean environments, using rigorous operational procedures (25), which adds significant cost and complexity to the manufacturing process.

Nonetheless, the small, shallow breaches from microneedles have been shown to pose low practical risk of infection (26). Manufacturers should assess risk to determine what level of bioburden control is appropriate for the clinical stage of development.

10.4 Biological Considerations

10.4.1 Biocompatibility

Microneedles have been produced from a wide range of materials, including metals, such as stainless steel or titanium, silicon, sugars, ceramics, non-degrading and degrading polymers, and hydrogels (27). Biocompatibility testing of the materials in their final, processed form is important to ensure that clinical products are acceptable for human exposure. Based on the guidelines for testing of surface devices on breached or compromised skin, Table 10.1 shows typical biocompatibility tests performed according to duration of skin contact (28).

TABLE 10.1

Guidelines for Biocompatibility Testing

Contact Duration with Skin	Recommended	Factors to Consider, Particularly for Degrading or Dissolving Materials, Which Increase Systemic Exposure
Limited: ≤24 h	• Cytotoxicity • Sensitization • Irritation or intracutaneous reactivity	• Acute systemic toxicity • Material-mediated pyrogenicity • Chemical characterization of extracted material
Prolonged: >24 h and ≤30 days	Same as limited	Same as limited, plus: • Subacute/subchronic systemic toxicity • Implantation
Chronic, repeated wear of the device: >30 days	Same as prolonged, plus: • Genotoxicity • Subacute/subchronic systemic toxicity	Same as prolonged, plus: • Chronic toxicity • Carcinogenicity

10.4.2 Irritation, Sensitization, and Immune Response

In addition to irritation from the microneedle, delivery of the active agent may irritate the skin (7). Skin irritation testing in an animal model of microneedle drug or vaccine delivery products is performed as a special toxicity test prior to human clinical testing (29). Human studies specifically focused on irritation and sensitization evaluation are performed during clinical development (30), and irritation and sensitization are also evaluated as part of the safety assessment during clinical trials.

The skin is a highly immunogenic organ, as one of its major functions is to protect the body from pathogenic organisms. Hence, the possibility of skin sensitization or even a systemic immune response (e.g., anaphylaxis) to microneedle delivery may be higher than for other routes of administration, such as subcutaneous injection. For drug delivery, this safety concern must be evaluated during animal testing prior to human studies, as well as during human clinical testing (31). For vaccines, the high immune responsiveness of the skin is a potential advantage of microneedle delivery, as a smaller, dose-sparing amount of vaccine may be sufficient to elicit the desired immune response (32).

10.4.3 Skin Healing

The skin rapidly detects a breach of its integrity and forms a rapid response to heal and seal the pores (33). For short duration systems, such as coated or dissolving microneedles (poke and remove) or intradermal injection (poke and push), rapid skin healing is a desirable process. It reduces the potential for infection and minimizes skin irritation. However, for applications that require longer durations of contact, such as pretreating the skin prior to patch placement (poke and place) or continuous delivery through hollow needles (poke and leave), skin healing closes the pathways and decreases delivery.

The needle dimensions (34), subject age (35), occlusion (36), and formulation of material that is placed against the skin (37) influence the rate of closure of skin pathways. An example is shown in Figure 10.1 (38). Hollow silicon microneedle arrays attached to a fluid-filled sampling chamber were worn by human subjects for periods ranging from six hours to three days. During study sessions, fluid was removed and replaced at 15-minute intervals and analyzed for glucose to determine the rate of glucose diffusion from the interstitial fluid in the skin through the needle lumens and compared to blood glucose obtained by finger-stick. The fluid was either phosphate-buffered saline (PBS) as a control or a proprietary formulation, compared side by side on each study subject. Photographs of the microneedles were taken over a light box before and after a three-day wear period. In Figure 10.1, the microneedle array and sampling chamber are shown. After use, the microneedle lumens were blocked for the PBS control (left), but remained open for three days using the proprietary formulation (right).

Figure 10.2 shows how the diffusion rate for glucose in the PBS (left) decreases with time relative to blood glucose over a six-hour wear period, whereas the proprietary formulation (right) maintains the relationship between blood glucose and the glucose diffusing through the lumens, indicating the transport pathway remained open. Glucose diffusion was close to zero at three days of wear in PBS, but continued for over three days of continuous wear with the proprietary formulation (data not shown).

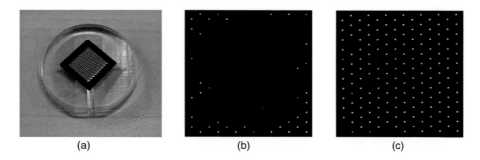

(a)   (b)   (c)

FIGURE 10.1   Microneedle array and sampling chamber (a). Backlit images of microneedle lumens after 72 hours of wear with (b) PBS and (c) proprietary formulation.

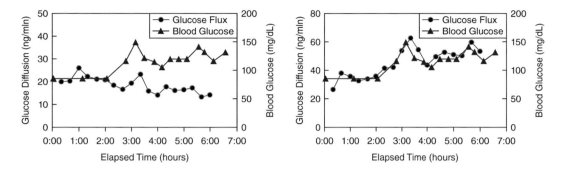

FIGURE 10.2 Glucose diffusion through hollow microneedles over six hours of wear in (left) phosphate-buffered saline and (right) proprietary formulation.

10.5 Procedural Requirements for Clinical Testing

10.5.1 Clinical Ethics Requirements

Sponsors, who initiate and manage clinical trials, and Investigators, who conduct clinical trials, must abide by ethical standards to ensure the safety and welfare of the clinical study subjects. Ethical requirements include performing studies according to clinical protocols, getting approval from institutional review boards (IRBs), and obtaining informed consent from study subjects to ensure they are aware of the risks of the study and are participating voluntarily (39–42). For drug or biologics studies beyond Phase I or medical device studies beyond small feasibility studies, registration on a clinical trials registry, such as clinicaltrials.gov, is an ethical responsibility to ensure that there is full disclosure of clinical data (43). For clinical studies intended for regulatory submission, Investigators must provide financial disclosure of potential conflicts of interest (44).

10.5.2 Regulatory Submissions for Microneedles for Clinical Studies

To engage in human clinical testing, manufacturers must document implementation of controls to ensure the benefit of the study exceeds its risks, typically through a submission to regulatory authorities. In the United States, for medical devices, the submission is an investigational device exemption (IDE) (45) and for drugs or vaccines it is an investigational new drug (IND) (29) application.

The submission for medical devices includes an IRB-approved clinical protocol and informed consent, reports of nonclinical safety testing (e.g., biocompatibility), manufacturing process controls (e.g., bioburden control), device design controls, and risk management. Studies investigating use of microneedles as devices (no active therapeutic agent) may qualify as nonsignificant risk studies (NSR) by submission of rationale to an IRB. If the IRB approves NSR status, submission of the IDE to FDA is not required, and documentation of abbreviated IDE controls is maintained by the Sponsor.

Microneedle drug or vaccine delivery products require IND submission prior to human clinical trials and include the content described above, plus animal data on drug absorption and pharmacokinetics or immune response by the microneedle route of administration, special local toxicity data on skin irritation, and a chemistry, manufacturing, and controls (CMC) report showing control over the composition, potency, purity, and manufacturing of the drug product (46, 47).

A significant development activity for both medical devices and combination products is design control (16, 48). Key elements to prepare for clinical studies include a design and development plan, design inputs, design outputs, design verification testing, and design reviews. Design inputs include specifications or requirements for the functionality (e.g., drug dose, sensor sensitivity), form (e.g., microneedle length), and safety (e.g., biocompatibility, bioburden specifications) of the product design. Design outputs are the results of the design process (e.g., product drawings, materials specifications). Design verification is demonstration that the design outputs meet the requirements of the design input, typically through *in vitro* or animal testing. Prior to human clinical testing, a formal design review evaluates the results of design verification testing to ensure the clinical product meets safety and functional requirements to be used on human subjects. Additionally, risk management is implemented to ensure controls are in place to minimize risk to the subjects (49). The clinical studies themselves, as well as human factors studies, are key elements of design validation to demonstrate that the product meets the user needs in the intended use environment.

10.6 Microneedle Applications with Human Clinical Experience

10.6.1 Cosmetic Applications

Cosmetic microneedle use can consist entirely of mechanical skin perturbation, with rollers or arrays of needles, for reduction of wrinkles, acne scars, and stretch marks, purportedly by increasing collagen production (50). Cosmetic use can also include skin pretreatment or microinjection to enable faster penetration of cosmetic agents, such as collagen creams or vitamin C (7). Some cosmetic devices are registered with FDA as Class I devices (510(k)-exempt), the lowest risk classification for medical devices. Class I devices cannot make therapeutic claims (e.g., "reduces wrinkles," "promotes collagen production") in promotional material, and needle lengths must be less than 0.3 mm (51). The regulatory barriers for cosmetic use have historically been minimal, but recently the FDA has issued warning letters to several manufacturers (52, 53) and has stated, "At this time [2015], the safe ranges of needle lengths, penetration depths, and speeds of the device are unknown; therefore, FDA has safety concerns regarding the potential for the needles to damage vessels and nerves." (54).

10.6.2 Sensing and Diagnostics

Microneedles can be used to painlessly access skin interstitial fluid, which has strong similarities to plasma, with comparable concentrations for many compounds (3). Collection of interstitial fluid from human subjects with offline analysis of analytes has been demonstrated with hydrogel microneedles for caffeine and glucose (55) and glass hollow microneedles for glucose (56). Clinical studies have demonstrated that interstitial fluid accessed by hollow microneedles coupled to an *in situ* electrochemical sensor can quantitatively measure blood glucose in diabetic subjects continuously over three days (57).

10.6.3 Drug Delivery

Local delivery of drugs to human subjects has been demonstrated for methyl nicotinate for vasodilation (58), lidocaine (59), and dyclonine (60) for numbing of the skin, and 5-aminolevulinate coupled with photodynamic therapy for treatment of basal cell carcinoma (61). Systemic delivery of naltrexone was one of the earliest clinical demonstrations of microneedle delivery (36). Studies of insulin delivery and pharmacokinetics have shown faster absorption by intradermal compared to subcutaneous injection (62–65). Several microneedle products are in clinical development toward commercialization. Zosano Pharma, Inc. has reported Phase III clinical trials of microneedles coated with zolmitriptan for migraine treatment (66), Phase II trials of human parathyroid hormone (PTH 1-34) (67) for osteoporosis treatment (68), and Phase II testing for glucagon for emergency hypoglycemia treatment (69). Corium has reported Phase II for a dissolving microneedle PTH formulation (70). Clearside Biomedical has used a single microneedle for delivery of corticosteroids to the eye for treatment of uveitis (71).

10.6.4 Vaccine Delivery

The Becton Dickinson Soluvia™ Micro Injection system, consisting of a single 1.5-mm stainless steel microneedle attached to a traditional syringe, is used in the commercial product Fluzone® intradermal influenza vaccine (7) and has been studied for rabies vaccination (72). NanoPass™ MicronJet600™ has

510(k) clearance and is CE-marked; it consists of three 600-micron-long silicon microneedles that can attach to a standard syringe. NanoPass microneedle devices have been used in human clinical studies to deliver vaccines for pandemic and seasonal strains of influenza (73), herpes zoster (74), and polio in infant populations (75), and in tuberculin skin testing (76). Dissolving microneedles have entered clinical testing for influenza vaccination (77, 78).

10.7 Conclusion

Microneedles are steadily progressing from laboratory research into clinical development to commercialization. Development can be a complex process, requiring an interdisciplinary approach, using chemistry, manufacturing, mechanical, and biological knowledge and capabilities. Additionally, regulatory and ethical requirements must be fulfilled before engaging in human clinical testing.

REFERENCES

1. Quinn HL, Kearney MC, Courtenay AJ et al. The role of microneedles for drug and vaccine delivery. Expert Opin Drug Deliv. 2014; 11(11): p. 1769–1780.
2. Kim YC, Park JH, Prausnitz MR. Microneedles for drug and vaccine delivery. Adv Drug Deliv Rev. 2012; 64(14): p. 1547–1568.
3. Romanyuk AV, Zvezdin VN, Samant P et al. Collection of analytes from microneedle patches. Anal Chem. 2014; 86(2): p. 10520–10523.
4. Prausnitz M. Microneedles for transdermal drug delivery. Adv Drug Delivery Rev. 2004; 56: p. 581–587.
5. FDA. The FDA's drug review process: Ensuring drugs are safe and effective. [Online]. [cited 2017 May 16]. Available from: https://www.fda.gov/Drugs/ResourcesForYou/Consumers/ucm143534.htm
6. Donnelly RF. Chapter 3: Microneedle applicator designs for transdermal drug delivery applications. In Donnelly R, Singh T, Morrow D, Woolfson A. Microneedle-mediated Transdermal and Intradermal Drug Delivery. Chichester, UK.: John Wiley & Sons, Ltd.; 2012.
7. Kalluri H, Choi S-O, Guo XD et al. Evaluation of microneedles in human subjects. In Dragicevic N, Maibach H. Percutaneous Penetration Enhancers Physical Methods in Penetration Enhancement. Berlin Heidelberg: Springer; 2017. p. 325–340.
8. Gupta J, Park S, Bondy B et al. Infusion pressure and pain during microneedle injection into skin of human subjects. Biomaterials. 2011; 32(28): p. 6823–6831.
9. Laurent PE, Bonnet S, Alchas P et al. Evaluation of the clinical performance of a new intradermal vaccine administration technique and associated delivery system. Vaccine. 2007; 25: p. 8833–8842.
10. Burton SA, Ng CY, Simmers R et al. Rapid intradermal delivery of liquid formulations using a hollow microstructured array. Pharm Res. 2011; 28(1): p. 31–40.
11. FDA Guidance. Applying human factors and usability engineering to medical devices. Feb 3, 2016.
12. FDA Guidance. Human factors studies and related clinical study considerations in combination product design and development draft guidance for industry and FDA staff. Feb 2016.
13. EN 62366-1. Medical devices—Part 1: Application of usability engineering to medical devices.
14. 21 CFR Part 211. Current good manufacturing practice for finished pharmaceuticals.
15. 21 CFR Parts 600–680. Biologics.
16. 21 CFR Part 820. Quality system regulation.
17. FDA Guidance. Current good manufacturing practice requirements for combination products. Jan 2017.
18. USP. Uniformity of dosage.
19. Ameri M, Fan SC, Maa YF. Parathyroid hormone PTH(1-34) formulation that enables uniform coating on a novel transdermal microprojection delivery system. Pharm Res. 2010; 27: p. 303–313.
20. ISO 14937. Sterilization of health care products. General requirements for characterization of a sterilizing agent and the development, validation and routine control of a sterilization process for medical devices. 2009.
21. FDA Guidance. Container and closure system integrity testing in lieu of sterility testing as a component of the stability protocol for sterile products. Feb 2008.
22. ISO 11607. Packaging for terminally sterilized medical devices. 2006.

23. McCrudden MTC, Alkila AZ, Courtenay AJ et al. Cosiderations in the sterile manufacture of polymeric microneedle arrays. Drug Deliv and Transl Res. 2015; 5: p. 3–14.
24. Ameri M, Wang X, Maa YF. Effect of irradiation on parathyroid hormone PTH(1-34) coated on a novel transdermal microprojection delivery system to produce a sterile product–adhesive compatibility. J Pharm Sci. 2010; 99(4): p. 2123–2134.
25. FDA Guidance. Sterile drug products produced by aseptic processing—Current good manufacturing practice. Sept 2004.
26. Donnelly RF, Singh TR, Tunney MM et al. Microneedle arrays allow lower microbial penetration than hypodermic needles in vitro. Pharm Res. 2009; 26(11): p. 2513–2522.
27. Larrañeta E, Lutton REM, Woolfson AD, Donnelly RF. Microneedle arrays as transdermal and intra-dermal drug delivery systems: Materials science, manufacture and commercial development. Mater Sci Eng R Rep. 2016; 104: p. 1–32.
28. FDA Guidance. Use of International Standard ISO 10993-1, "Biological evaluation of medical devices—Part 1: Evaluation and testing within a risk management process, FDA Guidance for Industry. Jun 16, 2016.
29. 21 CFR Part 312. IND content and format.
30. FDA Guidance. Skin irritation and sensitization testing of generic transdermal drug products. Dec 1999.
31. van der Maaden K, Jiskoot W, Bouwstra J. Microneedle technologies for (trans)dermal drug and vaccine delivery. J Controlled Release. 2012 July; 161(2): p. 645–655.
32. Prausnitz MR, Mikszta JS, Cormier M, Andrianov AK. Microneedle-based vaccines. Curr Top Microbiol Immunol. 2009; 333: p. 369–393.
33. Kalluri H, Banga AK. Formation and closure of microchannels in skin following microporation. Pharm Res. 2011; 28(1): p. 82–94.
34. Gupta J, Gill HS, Andres SN, Prausnitz MR. Kinetics of skin resealing after insertion of microneedles in human subjects. J. Control Release. 2011; 154(2): p. 148–155.
35. Kelchen MS, Siefers KJ, Converse CC et al. Micropore closure kinetics are delayed following microneedle insertion in elderly subjects. J. Control Release. 2016; 225: p. 294–300.
36. Wermeling DP, Banks SL, Hudson DA et al. Microneedles permit transdermal delivery of an impermeant medication to humans. PNAS. 2008; 105(6): p. 2058–2063.
37. Cormier M, Johnson J, Lin W et al. Inventors; Methods for inhibiting decrease in transdermal drug flux by inhibition of pathway closure. U.S. patent 7438926. Oct 21, 2008.
38. Tamada JA, Tierney MJ, Desai S et al. Design and evaluation of a MicroTip™ array-based continuous glucose monitor. In Presented at the 11th Annual Diabetes Technology Meeting; 2012; Bethesda, MD.
39. 21 CFR Part 50. Protection of human subjects.
40. 45 CFR Part 46. Subparts A, B, C, and D protection of humans.
41. ICH E6(R1). Good clinical practice: Consolidated guideline. 1996.
42. ISO 14155. Clinical investigation of medical devices for human subjects—Good clinical practice. 2011.
43. 42 CFR Part 11. Clinical trials registration and results information submission, final rule.
44. 21 CFR Part 54. Financial disclosure by clinical investigators.
45. 21 CFR Part 812. Investigational device exemptions.
46. FDA Guidance. Exploratory IND studies. Guidance for industry, investigators, and reviewers. 2006.
47. FDA Guidance. Content and format of investigational new drug applications (INDs) for phase 1 studies of drugs, including well-characterized, therapeutic, biotechnology-derived products.; Nov 1995.
48. ISO 13485. Medical devices—Quality management systems—Requirements for regulatory purposes. 2016.
49. ISO 14971. Medical devices—Application of risk management to medical Devices. 2007.
50. Majid I. Microneedling therapy in atrophic facial scars: An objective assessment. J Cutan Aesthet Surg. 2009; 2: p. 26–30.
51. Trow R. Rollers and the FDA: Fact vs. Fiction A regulatory update on a popular aesthetic trend. Modern Aesthetics. 2015 May/Jun: p. 46–47.
52. FDA Warning Letter. Bellus Medical 9/13/16.; Sep 13, 2016. Available from: https://www.fda.gov/iceci/enforcementactions/warningletters/2016/ucm520649.htm
53. FDA Warning Letter. Cynergy, LLC/Dermaroller Gmbh 3/1/13. Mar 1, 2013. Available from: https://www.fda.gov/ICECI/EnforcementActions/WarningLetters/ucm342779.htm

54. FDA Warning Letter. Derma Pen, LLC 1/9/15. Jan 9, 2015. Available from: https://www.fda.gov/iceci/enforcementactions/warningletters/2015/ucm429899.htm

55. Caffarel-Salvador E, Brady AJ, Eltayib E et al. Hydrogel-forming microneedle arrays allow detection of drugs and glucose in vivo: potential for use in diagnosis and therapeutic drug monitoring [10.1371/journal.pone.0145644]; 2015.

56. Wang PM, Cornwell M, Prausnitz MR. Minimally invasive extraction of dermal interstitial fluid for glucose monitoring using micronedles. Diabetes Technol Ther. 2005; 7(1): p. 131–141.

57. Jina A, Tierney MJ, Tamada JA et al. Design, development, and evaluation of a novel microneedle array-based continuous glucose monitor. Diabetes Technol Thera. 2014; 8(3): p. 483–487.

58. Sivamani RK, Stoeber B, Wu GC et al. Clinical microneedle injection of methyl nicotinate: Stratum corneum penetration. Skin Res Technol. 2005; 11(2): p. 152–156.

59. Gupta J, Denson DD, Felner EI, Prausnitz MR. Rapid local anesthesia in human subjects using minimally invasive microneedles. Clin J Pain. 2012; 28(2): p. 129–135.

60. Li X, Zhao R, Qin Z et al. Microneedle pretreatment improves efficacy of cutaneous topical anesthesia. Am J Emerg Med. 2010; 28: p. 130–134.

61. Mikolajewska P, Donnelly RF, Garlad MJ et al. Microneedle pre-treatment of human skin improves 5-aminolevulinic acid (ALA)- and 5- aminolevulinic acid methy ester (MAL)-induced PpIX production for topical photodynamic therapy without increase in pain or erythema. Pharm Res. 2010; 27(10): p. 2213–2220.

62. Gupta J, Felner EI, Prausnitz MR. Rapid pharmacokinetics of intradermal insulin administered. Diabetes Tech Thera. 2011; 13(4): p.451-456.

63. Rini CJ, McVey E, Sutter D et al. Intradermal insulin infusion achieves faster insulin action than subcutaneous infusion for 3-day wear. Drug Deliv Transl Res. 2015; 5: p. 332–345.

64. Pettis RJ, Hirsch L, Kapitza C et al. Microneedle-based intradermal versus subcutaneous administration of regular human insulin or insulin lispro: pharmacokinetics and postprandial glycemic excursions in patients with type 1 diabetes. Diabetes Technol Ther. 2011 Apr; 13(4): p. 443.

65. Kochba E, Levin Y, Raz I, Cahn A. Improved insulin pharmacokinetics using a novel microneedle device for intradermal delivery in patients with type 2 diabetes. Diabetes Technol Thera. 2016; 18(9): p. 525–531.

66. Zosano Pharma, Inc. Zosano Pharma announces 3.8 mg Dose of M207, its novel transdermal therapeutic, meets both co-primary endpoints in the ZOTRIP Pivotal efficacy trial in migraine. [Online]; Feb 13, 2017 [2017 May 20 date accesssed]. Available from: http://ir.zosanopharma.com/releasedetail.cfm?ReleaseID=1011563

67. Daddona PE, Matriano JA, Mandema J, Maa YF. Parathyroid hormone (1-34)-coated microneedle patch system: clinical pharmacokinetics and pharmacodynamics for treatment of osteoporosis. Pharm Res. 2010; p. 159–165.

68. Cosman FN, Lane E, Bolognese MA et al. Effect of transdermal teriparatide administration on bone mineral density in postmenopausal women. J Clin Endocrinol Metab. 2010; 95: p. 151–158.

69. Zosano Pharma, Inc. Zosano Pharma announces positive phase 2 results for its ZP-Glucagon Patch Program for treatment of severe hypoglycemia. [Online]; Oct 13, 2015 [May20, 2017 date accessed]. Available from: http://ir.zosanopharma.com/releasedetail.cfm?releaseid=936338

70. Corium International, Inc. Corium announces positive topline results from phase 2a study of transdermal MicroCor(R) PTH in post-menopausal women. [Online]; Jul 28, 2015. Available from: http://ir.coriumgroup.com/releasedetail.cfm?releaseid=924281

71. Goldstein DA, Do D, Noronha G et al. Suprachoroidal corticosteroid administration: Aa novel route for local treatment of noninfectious uveitis. Trans. Vis. Sci. Tech. 2016; 5(6): p. 14.

72. Laurent PE, Bourhy H, Fantino M et al. Safety and efficacy of novel dermal and epidermal microneedle delivery systems for rabies vaccination in healthy adults. Vaccine. 2010; 28(36): p. 5850–5856.

73. Levin Y, Kochba E, Hung I, Kenney R. Intradermal vaccination using the novel. Hum Vaccin Immunother. 2015 April; 11(4): p. 991–997.

74. Beals CR, Raikar RA, Schaeffer AK et al. Immune response and reactogenicity of intradermal administration versus subcutaneous administration of varicella-zoster virus vaccine: an exploratory, randomised, partly blinded trial. Lancet Infect Dis. 2016 August; 16(8): p. 915–922.

75. Anand A, Zaman K, Estívariz CF et al. Early priming with inactivated poliovirus vaccine (IPV) and intradermal fractional dose IPV administered by a microneedle device: A randomized controlled trial. Vaccine. 2015; 33(48): p. 6816–6822.
76. Lee HJ, Choi HJ, Kim DR et al. Safety and efficacy of tuberculin skin testing with microneedle MicronJet600(TM) in healthy adults. Int J Tuberc Lung Dis. 2016; 20(4): p. 500–504.
77. Hirobe S, Azukizawa H, Hanafusa T et al. Clinical study and stability assessment of a novel transcutaneanous influenze vaccination using a dssvoling microneedle patch. BIomaterials. 2015; 57: p. 50–58.
78. Prausnitz M. Inactivated influenza vaccine delivered by microneedle patch or by hypodermic needle. [Online]. [cited 2017 May 29]. Available from: https://clinicaltrials.gov/ct2/show/NCT02438423

11

Microneedling in Clinical Practice

Cosmetic applications

Aunna Pourang, MD
Kourosh Beroukhim, MD
University of California-Davis

11.1 Introduction

The demand for effective, minimally invasive esthetic procedures is on the rise. There was a 186% increase in the number of minimally invasive cosmetic procedures performed between 2000 and 2017, as opposed to a 6% overall decrease in cosmetic surgical procedures in the same period (1). Microneedling is an effective, relatively safe, minimally invasive procedure that has been shown to rejuvenate the skin, improve scars, rhytides, and striae and provide other esthetic enhancements with limited side effects and post-procedure recovery time.

11.2 The Origins of Microneedling

While the scope of microneedling has expanded beyond cosmetic purposes to include various medical uses, the technology is rooted in the field of esthetics. Early in the development of needling procedures, several groups reported using needles to undermine depressed scars by cutting through the fibrous tissue and creating a space to inject various dermal filler agents (2, 3). Orentreich and Orentreich developed the subcision technique, a subcuticular undermining technique using a hypodermic needle, for depressed cutaneous scars and wrinkles (4). Camirand and Doucet incidentally noticed an improvement in the appearance of hypochromic scars that were previously tattooed. They eventually developed a technique using needle microdermabrasion to repigment and soften scars (5). Based on these concepts, Fernandes developed a rolling needle device that allowed sufficient dermal penetration to stimulate collagen production (6). Shortly after, Liebl patented the Dermaroller™ device (7). Since then many different types of microneedling devices, ranging from home care rollers to automated pens, have been developed to meet the increasing demands of anti-aging procedures.

11.3 The Biology of Aging Skin

The cutaneous aging process involves both intrinsic and extrinsic mechanisms, with the former involving mostly genetic factors and the latter comprising external factors such as the sun, smoking, and poor nutrition (8). On a histological level, intrinsically aged skin shows dermal and epidermal atrophy, flattening of rete ridges, reduced fibroblasts, fragmented collagen bundles, increased number of collagen fibrils, and increased ratio of collagen III to collagen I in the dermis (9–11). On a grosser level, these changes manifest as thin, sagging skin with exaggerated expression lines and the loss of subcutaneous volume. Similar, yet more pronounced histologic changes are noted in extrinsically aged skin, in addition to the presence of elastosis and hyperpigmented lesions caused by UV light exposure (8). Aging skin, in general, may be dryer and rougher with increased pallor due to decreased vasculature.

While the avoidance of exposure to extrinsic factors is key to prevention, several treatments are available for rejuvenating aging skin. Treatments are often geared to resurfacing the epidermis and replacing dermal volume loss. The result is youthful-appearing skin that is smooth, tight, plump, hydrated, and wrinkle- and blemish-free.

Although lasers, chemical peels, and microdermabrasion are effective treatments, their mechanism of action involves destruction of the epidermis, which leads to an inflammatory response, subsequently producing new collagen. This mechanism also has the potential to induce post-inflammatory hyperpigmentation (12–14). Although the dermal fibrosis produced by ablative therapies can lead to skin tightening, there is an increased risk of scarring in addition to disordered collagen formation (15–17). Microneedling, on the other hand, can produce similar cosmetic results with decreased risk of hyperpigmentation, pain, erythema, and short recovery downtime (18).

11.4 Mechanism of Action

Microneedling induces minimal epidermal injury, mitigating the adverse effects seen with ablative therapies. In fact, re-epithelialization occurs within 24 hours and epidermal barrier function is, for the most part, maintained (19, 20). The main postulated mechanism by which microneedling confers most of its benefits is through collagen induction that occurs during the body's normal response to trauma and wound healing. For this reason, microneedling is often referred to as percutaneous collagen induction therapy.

Microneedling devices deliver several micropuncture wounds to the skin, activating the three-step wound healing response – inflammation, proliferation, and remodeling – ultimately resulting in dermal collagen formation. This results in thicker skin with increased collagen deposition in a normal lattice design, increased elastin content, epidermal thickening, and normal rete ridges (21–23). Clinically significant results may not be seen for several weeks after treatment, with maximal effects noted at 12–24 weeks and continued changes for up to 8–12 months (24, 25).

It is hypothesized that the controlled wound milieu, as a result of minimal stress and decreased exposure to infection, enables regeneration of normal tissue and avoids scar tissue formation (26). Since the basement membrane is not damaged and the inflammatory response does not affect epidermal melanocytes, pigmentation issues do not typically occur, as they do in deep chemical peels, dermabrasion, and lasers (22, 25–27). Microarray analysis has identified an upregulation of genes associated with tissue remodeling and wound healing, and a downregulation of pro-inflammatory cytokines associated with microneedling of in vitro skin models (28).

Another proposed mechanism by which microneedling induces collagen formation is the theory of bioelectricity. The fine wounds caused by needling causes cells to react with a demarcation current that is increased by the needles' electrical potential. The change in electric potential in the cell membrane creates increased cell activity, release of potassium ions, proteins, and growth factors. The body is fooled into believing an injury has occurred and, through an unclear mechanism, new collagen deposition results in the upper dermis (29).

Microneedling is also used as a transdermal drug delivery system which may account for the enhanced effectiveness of topical agents used for various cosmetic applications, such as the treatment of melasma and alopecia (30, 31).

11.5 Indications

11.5.1 Anti-Aging

Microneedling is effective for skin rejuvenation by way of neocollagenesis. Many studies have demonstrated the improvement of rhytides, skin thickness, skin irregularity, skin texture, and skin laxity on the face, neck, abdomen, and other parts of the body with microneedling treatments (23, 25, 32–34).

In treating photodamage and actinic keratoses using microneedling followed by photodynamic therapy with either aminolevulonic acid or methyl aminolevulinate, patients found an improvement in global photoaging, roughness, sallowness, fine lines, and mottled pigmentation (35, 36).

While the face is a common site for treatments, other areas of the body such as the neck, abdomen, arms, thighs, and the between the breasts can also be treated (6).

11.5.2 Scars

Several studies have demonstrated the beneficial effects of microneedling on acne scars (37). Rolling and boxcar scars respond well to microneedling treatment as opposed to deep or icepick scars, with a corresponding increase in types I, III, VII, and newly synthesized collagen as well as tropoelastin (38). Fractional radiofrequency microneedling, on the other hand, has been shown to improve icepick acne scars (39). Hypertrophic scars and keloids have shown improvement in combination therapy with silicone gel (40). Silicone gel is thought to improve scars by increasing hydration of the stratum corneum, with subsequent cytokine-mediated signaling from keratinocytes to dermal fibroblasts to downregulate extracellular matrix production (41). Microneedling's synergistic action of collagen remodeling likely accounts for the improvement seen in this combination.

Aust et al. demonstrated an improvement in post-burn scars with microneedling treatments in addition to pre-procedural and post-procedural topical application of vitamins A and C (27). Histological exams showed a normalization of the collagen and elastin matrix in the reticular dermis, and an increase in collagen deposition at 12 months, postoperatively. The collagen appeared to have been laid down in a normal lattice pattern, rather than the parallel bundles seen in scar tissue. An improvement in posttraumatic scars, post-varicella scars, and post-herpetic scars has also been noted with microneedling treatments (42–44). Striae distensae, a form of scarring, has also shown statistically significant improvement with microneedling (22, 45, 46).

11.5.3 Pigmentary Disorders

Pigmentation disorders respond well to microneedling when combined with other therapies. Studies have shown an improvement in melasma in conjunction with topical agents, including tranexamic acid, as well as a depigmentation serum containing rucinol and sophora-alpha and another containing 0.05% tretinoin, 4% hydroquinone, and 1% flucinonide acetonide (30, 47, 48). A case of severe, idiopathic periorbital melanosis improved with lightening and anti-aging serums and a DermaFrac device (Genesis Biosystems, Lewisville, TX), which combines microneedling using precisely calibrated needle penetration with simultaneous vacuum-assisted serum infusion (49). Similar outcomes were seen using microneedling following 10% trichloroacetic acid peels for periorbital melanosis (50). The efficacy in the treatment of vitiligo is limited and further studies using microneedling as a transdermal drug delivery method are necessary (51, 52).

11.5.4 Alopecia

Dhurat et al. have demonstrated an improvement in androgenetic alopecia using both microneedling with 5% minoxidil and microneedling without a topical medication in individuals who continued to take their routine minoxidil and finasteride (53, 54). The authors postulated that in addition to the release of growth factors seen in wound healing, microneedling also stimulates stem cells in the hair bulge as a result of the wound healing cascade. Microneedling is also thought to stimulate the expression of hair growth-related genes (55–57). Cases of alopecia areata have also improved with microneedling followed by triamcinolone acetonide, likely as a result of enhanced transdermal drug delivery (31).

11.6 Combined Therapies

Microneedling can enhance other rejuvenation modalities while minimizing complications associated with more abrasive interventions.

11.6.1 Peels

Thirty-five percent glycolic acid peel performed 3 weeks after microneedling was shown to enhance acne scar improvement and post-inflammatory hyperpigmentation when compared to microneedling alone (58). Microneedling combined with 20% trichloroacetic acid peel creates results similar to a deep phenol peel and non-ablative fractional lasers with significantly less duration of post-procedural erythema (59, 60).

11.6.2 Subcision

Microneedling and subcision of acne scars demonstrated efficacy in 100% of patients as opposed to 77% who received microneedling alone (61).

11.6.3 Fillers

Subdermal injections of 1:1 diluted calcium hydroxyapatite (Radiesse®) filler combined with microneedling and topical vitamin C improved stretch marks. This combination was also shown to increase the quantity and quality of collagen and elastin fibers in treated areas compared to untreated skin and areas treated with microneedling and ascorbic acid alone (62).

11.6.4 Platelet-Rich Plasma

Platelet-rich plasma (PRP) contains multiple autologous growth factors, such as epidermal growth factor, platelet-derived growth factor, transforming growth factor-β, vascular endothelial growth factor, fibroblast growth factor, and more. Not only does microneedling enhance PRP absorption in the skin, but the growth factors found in PRP act synergistically with growth factors induced by skin needling to enhance the wound-healing response (63, 64).

PRP with microneedling has been shown to improve acne scars more than microneedling alone with results similar to intradermal PRP and 100% topical trichloroacetic acid (TCA) (65, 66).

11.6.5 Stem Cells

Stem cell therapy has been shown to have benefits in skin rejuvenation therapy (67–69). Like PRP, endothelial precursor cells (EPCs) differentiated from human embryonic stem cells (hESCs) also contain growth factors and cytokines, which have been shown to improve blood perfusion in damaged tissues (70–72). Conditioned medium of hESC-derived EPCs has been shown to significantly improve the proliferation and migration of dermal fibroblasts and epidermal keratinocytes and increase collagen synthesis in fibroblasts (70). Microneedling is used with stem cell therapy to enhance penetration through the stratum corneum and has been found to improve pigmentation and wrinkles more than microneedling alone (73).

11.6.6 Topical Agents

Topical serums are often used during microneedling procedures as lubricants to minimize skin abrasion. Some authors believe that the use of vitamins A and C is important given their importance in skin health, in particular their roles in collagen regeneration and formation (6, 22, 74–79). There have been reports of foreign-body granuloma reactions in individuals receiving microneedling treatments with topical vitamin C. Subsequent patch testing in these individuals revealed reactivity to vitamin C. It is thought that hypersensitivity reactions can occur with the application of topical products prior to microneedling via immunogenic particle absorption in the dermis (80). It is important that patients using a home microneedling device be educated on using only approved topical agents. There are different topical anti-aging regimens on the market that can be used before and after treatments (81).

11.7 Microneedling Devices

Several different types of microneedling devices exist. A standard dermaroller consists of a handle, attached to a single-use cylinder 2 cm in diameter and 2 cm wide, with 8 rows of microneedles around its circumference and 24 arrays of microneedles along its width. A total of 192 needles between 0.5 mm and 1.5 mm in length and 0.1 mm in diameter can be found in such a device. Fifteen passes over an area using a dermaroller with 192 needles 2 mm in length and 0.07 mm in diameter results in about 250 micropunctures/cm^2 (82). There are home care dermarollers on the market with needles less than 0.15 mm in length which are used for the transdermal delivery of anti-aging products (82). Tram-track scarring has been reported with the use of manual microneedling devices. It is recommended that gentle pressure and shorter needles be used over bony prominences and areas with thin skin when using these devices (83, 84).

Stamps are a modified version of the dermaroller with needles of 2 mm in length and 0.12 mm in diameter used for the treatment of hard-to-reach areas such as the upper lip or localized scars such as varicella scars (82, 85).

Automated microneedling devices typically contain a disposable tip with needles that operate at different speeds in a vibrating stamp-like manner, with the ability to adjust needle length as needed. The benefits of this device include convenience in treating narrow areas such as the nose and around the eyes, consistent depth of penetration, ergonomic benefits of automation, and the ability to use the same device every time (85, 86). Splashback has occurred in older devices, but newer devices have addressed this issue. DermaFrac™ (Genesis Biosystems) technology combines microneedling with simultaneous infusion of a serum with active ingredients (49).

Fractional radiofrequency microneedle (FRM) devices contain a disposable tip with gold-plated insulated needles which penetrate the skin and release radiofrequency currents through the dermis. The resultant heat induces neocollagenesis and neoelastogenesis. Needle depth, power, and duration of energy pulse can be adjusted. This technology is safe in darker skin types, because it does not damage the epidermis and has been shown to be effective at improving acne scars, aging skin, and enlarged pores (87–90). The FRM has been shown to decrease NF-κβ, IL-8, and sebum excretion rates, and to improve acne. Additionally, the increase of TGF-β1, TGF-β3, and collagen associated with FRM technology is thought to be the reason for acne scar improvement, as transforming growth factor activates dermal fibroblasts and enhances collagen formation (39).

11.8 Technique

Microneedling is a simple and effective tool that can be provided to patients in an esthetic medical practice. Figures 11.1–11.4 depict various aspects of a microneedling treatment session.

11.8.1 Considerations

There are several absolute contraindications to consider in individuals undergoing microneedling treatment. They include:

- Presence of skin cancers, herpes, or any other active skin infections
- Tendency to develop severe keloids
- Uncontrolled diabetes mellitus
- Presence of blood dyscrasias
- Genetic conditions with aberrant collagen deposition
- Patients on chemotherapy, radiation, high doses of corticosteroids, or medications that impede wound healing
- Metal allergy depending on the metal used for the microneedle (91)
- Hypersensitivity to topical agents

While concomitant botulinum toxin injections are not an absolute contraindication to microneedling treatments, care should be taken when microneedling recently injected sites, to avoid toxin diffusion. See below for further recommendations relating to performing multiple esthetic procedures in one sitting. Although there is a low risk of dyspigmentation with microneedling, treatment would benefit from being delayed if there is recent sun exposure to avoid post-treatment dyspigmentation. There are no established recommendations for herpes prophylaxis. However it is important to discuss the risks and have a preventive plan in place for patients with a history of facial herpes. Authors have varying opinions on whether to perform microneedling treatments in individuals who are on anti-coagulant therapies (6, 92). No studies have been done on this population, and as with any trauma in these individuals there is increased risk of bruising and bleeding.

11.8.2 Pretreatment

A thorough history and focused assessment of the treatment area should be undertaken, making sure to note the esthetic qualities of the skin.

Patients do not need to discontinue home skin care treatments prior to microneedling treatments. Recent treatments such as chemical peels, lasers, or dermal fillers do not preclude microneedling treatments, although clinical judgment should be used to determine whether the patient will be able to tolerate a second procedure. If multiple treatments are to be done on the same day, it is recommended that treatments be done in the order of deep-to-superficial layers of the skin. For example, dermal fillers should be done prior to a microneedling procedure to ensure landmarks remain visible and to prevent diffusion of injectables (92).

Standard steps for informed consent should be taken prior to beginning the procedure. As with any cosmetic treatment, it is important to take baseline and post-treatment photographs to demonstrate outcomes and assist with patient satisfaction.

Clean off any makeup from the skin and apply a nonoccluded compounded lidocaine 30% cream to the treatment area for about 20–30 minutes. Remove the anesthetic cream with water-soaked gauze and alcohol wipes.

11.8.3 Treatment

The following instructions apply to automated microneedling devices. It is important to be familiar with the manufacturer's recommendations regarding the speed and needle depth to be used for various locations. Needle depth should be adjusted based on skin thickness in the area being treated. For scars, striae, and areas with thicker skin such as the cheeks, needle depths of 1.5–3.0 mm may be used. In more delicate areas such as forehead, nasal bridge, and lower eyelids, needle depths of

0.5–1.0 mm may be used. Studies have shown that needle penetration matched settings up to 1.0 mm but were less consistent once needle lengths were longer than 1.0 mm (93, 94). Another study showed that the benefits of singular microneedling sessions with a 3 mm needle could be achieved by a singular treatment using a 1 mm needle size, which could be augmented further by repeating the treatment (95).

A topical agent is advised to maximize the glide of needles over the skin. Oftentimes, the manufacturer will provide a prepared agent, usually containing a mix of hyaluronic acid and antioxidants. Sterile, inert, water-based gels, and PRP can also be used.

Begin by ensuring there is a brand-new disposable needle cartridge in place. Apply the chosen topical agent to the skin in an adequate amount to minimize epidermal injury. Lower the device so that the needles are perpendicular to the skin while providing mild traction nearby with a free hand, taking care not to inflict a needlestick injury. Glide the device over the skin in all directions (horizontal, vertical, oblique) until pinpoint bleeding is visible, which usually occurs after 3–6 passes depending on the area treated. It may be helpful to treat thicker, less sensitive areas first to allow the patient to adjust to the pain he or she may experience. Once the procedure is complete, remove blood and the topical agent with sterile water-soaked gauze. Apply a post-procedure serum, also often provided by the manufacturer, to the treatment areas. Cooling masks without active ingredients may also be used to soothe any pain and swelling.

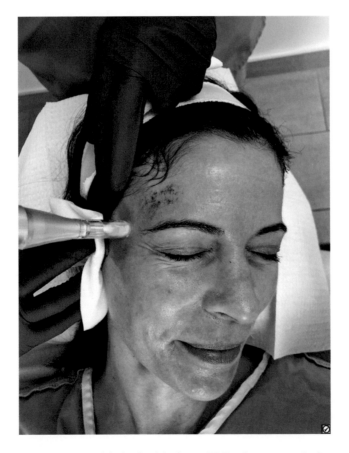

FIGURE 11.1 Microneedling treatment with platelet rich plasma (PRP) using automated microneedling pen. Note how the pen is held perpendicular to the skin while the other hand is used to hold traction at a safe distance from the pen. (Photo courtesy of Naissan Wesley, MD.)

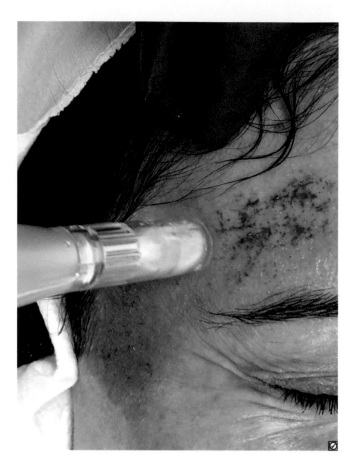

FIGURE 11.2   Closeup of microneedling treatment with PRP using automated microneedling pen. Uniform pinpoint bleeding is used as the endpoint of the treatment. (Photo courtesy of Naissan Wesley, MD.)

11.8.4 Post-Procedure

Patients may be supplied with a chosen topical serum to apply to their face for a few hours after the procedure. After 4 hours the patient can apply nonallergenic moisturizing cream 3 times a day for about 3 days. It is important to emphasize the importance of applying a nonchemical sunscreen with SPF 30 in addition to the moisturizer. Makeup can be applied 2 days after treatment but active skin care products should be resumed 1 week after treatment (92).

11.8.5 Number of Treatments

While there is no standard treatment protocol available, the literature shows time intervals between two sessions vary from 4 to 8 weeks with a total number of 2 to 4 treatment sessions (83). An animal study demonstrated that the best results are achieved when microneedling treatments are repeated 4 times with an interval time of 3 weeks (95). Starting off with 1 session every 2 to 4 weeks for a total of 3 sessions is a good place to start. It is also important to keep in mind that maximal effects may not appear for several months.

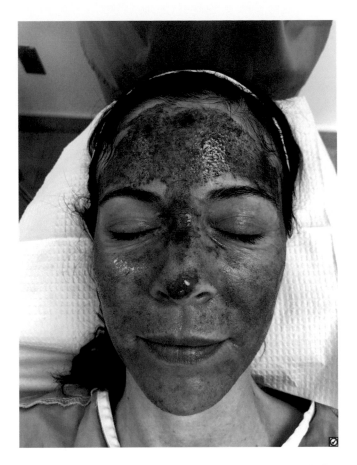

FIGURE 11.3 After microneedling treatment with PRP of the face using an automated microneedling pen. Note the uniform pinpoint bleeding. (Photo courtesy of Naissan Wesley, MD.)

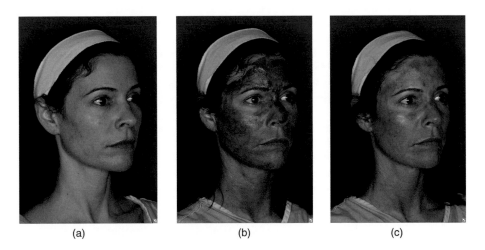

(a) (b) (c)

FIGURE 11.4 Photos of patient. **(a)** Before microneedling. **(b)** Immediately after microneedling of the face and neck with PRP. **(c)** After microneedling procedure with blood and PRP removed. The inflammation typically resolves within 24 hours. (Photos courtesy of Naissan Wesley, MD.)

TABLE 11.1

The Benefits and Disadvantages of Microneedling Treatments

Benefits	Disadvantages
• Decreased risk of hyperpigmentation, particularly with strict UV-light avoidance before and after the procedure • Short healing phase and minimal downtime • Can be performed on areas where lasers or peels cannot • Does not ablate the epidermis • More cost-effective than laser treatments • Excellent safety profile in all skin types • Low risk of infection when performed under sterile conditions and with appropriate post-procedural care (24).	• Pain, swelling, and erythema can occur • Bleeding can pose a risk to the provider and discomfort for the patient • Results may not initially be as impressive as those achieved with laser resurfacing • Scarring can occur if performed too aggressively • Potential increased risk of hypersensitivity reactions to topicals or needles

11.9 Conclusion

Microneedling is an innovative procedure that is helping meet the increased demand for non-surgical esthetic enhancement. Through a controlled wound healing cascade as a result of micropunctures, new collagen is formed, leading to improvement in rhytides and overall skin appearance. In addition to its anti-aging benefits, microneedling is also effective in treating scars, striae, melasma, and alopecia. When it is combined with other modalities such as PRP, dermal filler agents, and peels, esthetic results are enhanced. As a cost-effective, easily implementable in-office procedure, microneedling can provide esthetic benefits similar to those of peels and lasers with fewer side effects and minimal down time (Table 11.1).

REFERENCES

1. 2017 Complete Plastic Surgery Statistics Report: American Society of Plastic Surgeons. Available from: https://www.plasticsurgery.org/documents/News/Statistics/2017/plastic-surgery-statistics-full-report-2017.pdf
2. Spangler AS. New treatment for pitted scars; preliminary report. AMA Arch Derm. 1957;76(6):708–11.
3. Hambley RM, Carruthers JA. Microlipoinjection for the elevation of depressed full-thickness skin grafts on the nose. J Dermatol Surg Oncol. 1992;18(11):963–8.
4. Orentreich DS, Orentreich N. Subcutaneous incisionless (subcision) surgery for the correction of depressed scars and wrinkles. Dermatol Surg. 1995;21(6):543–9.
5. Camirand A, Doucet J. Needle dermabrasion. Aesthetic Plast Surg. 1997;21(1):48–51.
6. Fernandes D. Minimally invasive percutaneous collagen induction. Oral Maxillofac Surg Clin North Am. 2005;17(1):51–63, vi.
7. DERMAROLLER—Trademark Details: JUSTIA Trademarks. Available from: https://trademarks.justia.com/770/73/dermaroller-77073555.html
8. Baumann L. Skin ageing and its treatment. J Pathol. 2007;211(2):241–51.
9. Lovell CR, Smolenski KA, Duance VC, Light ND, Young S, Dyson M. Type I and III collagen content and fibre distribution in normal human skin during ageing. Br J Dermatol. 1987;117(4):419–28.
10. Fenske NA, Lober CW. Structural and functional changes of normal aging skin. J Am Acad Dermatol. 1986;15(4 Pt 1):571–85.
11. Roupe G. Skin of the aging human being. Lakartidningen. 2001;98(10):1091–5.
12. Dover JS, Hruza GJ. Laser skin resurfacing. Semin Cutan Med Surg. 1996;15(3):177–88.
13. Fulton JE, Porumb S. Chemical peels: their place within the range of resurfacing techniques. Am J Clin Dermatol. 2004;5(3):179–87.
14. Nelson BR, Fader DJ, Gillard M, Majmudar G, Johnson TM. Pilot histologic and ultrastructural study of the effects of medium-depth chemical facial peels on dermal collagen in patients with actinically damaged skin. J Am Acad Dermatol. 1995;32(3):472–8.

15. Wind BS, Meesters AA, Kroon MW, Beek JF, van der Veen JP, van der Wal AC, et al. Formation of fibrosis after nonablative and ablative fractional laser therapy. Dermatol Surg. 2012;38(3):437–42.

16. Fulton JE, Jr., Barnes T. Collagen shrinkage (selective dermaplasty) with the high-energy pulsed carbon dioxide laser. Dermatol Surg. 1998;24(1):37–41.

17. Fitzpatrick RE, Goldman MP, Satur NM, Tope WD. Pulsed carbon dioxide laser resurfacing of photo-aged facial skin. Arch Dermatol. 1996;132(4):395–402.

18. Leheta T, El Tawdy A, Abdel Hay R, Farid S. Percutaneous collagen induction versus full-concentration trichloroacetic acid in the treatment of atrophic acne scars. Dermatol Surg. 2011;37(2):207–16.

19. Donnelly RF, Raj Singh TR, Woolfson AD. Microneedle-based drug delivery systems: microfabrication, drug delivery, and safety. Drug Deliv. 2010;17(4):187–207.

20. Kalluri H, Kolli CS, Banga AK. Characterization of microchannels created by metal microneedles: formation and closure. AAPS J. 2011;13(3):473–81.

21. Velnar T, Bailey T, Smrkolj V. The wound healing process: an overview of the cellular and molecular mechanisms. J Int Med Res. 2009;37(5):1528–42.

22. Aust MC, Fernandes D, Kolokythas P, Kaplan HM, Vogt PM. Percutaneous collagen induction therapy: an alternative treatment for scars, wrinkles, and skin laxity. Plast Reconstr Surg. 2008;121(4):1421–9.

23. Fabbrocini G, Fardella N, Monfrecola A, Proietti I, Innocenzi D. Acne scarring treatment using skin needling. Clin Exp Dermatol. 2009;34(8):874–9.

24. Ramaut L, Hoeksema H, Pirayesh A, Stillaert F, Monstrey S. Microneedling: Where do we stand now? A systematic review of the literature. J Plast Reconstr Aesthet Surg. 2018;71(1):1–14.

25. Fabbrocini G, De Vita V, Monfrecola A, De Padova MP, Brazzini B, Teixeira F, et al. Percutaneous collagen induction: an effective and safe treatment for post-acne scarring in different skin phototypes. J Dermatolog Treat. 2014;25(2):147–52.

26. Aust MC, Reimers K, Repenning C, Stahl F, Jahn S, Guggenheim M, et al. Percutaneous collagen induction: minimally invasive skin rejuvenation without risk of hyperpigmentation-fact or fiction? Plast Reconstr Surg. 2008;122(5):1553–63.

27. Aust MC, Knobloch K, Reimers K, Redeker J, Ipaktchi R, Altintas MA, et al. Percutaneous collagen induction therapy: an alternative treatment for burn scars. Burns. 2010;36(6):836–43.

28. Schmitt L, Marquardt Y, Amann P, Heise R, Huth L, Wagner-Schiffler S, et al. Comprehensive molecular characterization of microneedling therapy in a human three-dimensional skin model. PLoS One. 2018;13(9):e0204318.

29. Liebl H, Kloth LC. Skin cell proliferation stimulated by microneedles. J Am Coll Clin Wound Spec. 2012;4(1):2–6.

30. Budamakuntla L, Loganathan E, Suresh DH, Shanmugam S, Suryanarayan S, Dongare A, et al. A randomised, open-label, comparative study of tranexamic acid microinjections and tranexamic acid with microneedling in patients with melasma. J Cutan Aesthet Surg. 2013;6(3):139–43.

31. Chandrashekar B, Yepuri V, Mysore V. Alopecia areata-successful outcome with microneedling and triamcinolone acetonide. J Cutan Aesthet Surg. 2014;7(1):63–4.

32. Fabbrocini G, De Vita V, Pastore F, Annunziata MC, Cacciapuoti S, Monfrecola A, et al. Collagen induction therapy for the treatment of upper lip wrinkles. J Dermatolog Treat. 2012;23(2):144–52.

33. Fabbrocini G, De Vita V, Di Costanzo L, Pastore F, Mauriello MC, Ambra M, et al. Skin needling in the treatment of the aging neck. Skinmed. 2011;9(6):347–51.

34. Ablon G. Safety and effectiveness of an automated microneedling device in improving the signs of aging skin. J Clin Aesthet Dermatol. 2018;11(8):29–34.

35. Clementoni MT, M BR, Munavalli GS. Photodynamic photorejuvenation of the face with a combination of microneedling, red light, and broadband pulsed light. Lasers Surg Med. 2010;42(2):150–9.

36. Torezan L, Chaves Y, Niwa A, Sanches JA, Jr., Festa-Neto C, Szeimies RM. A pilot split-face study comparing conventional methyl aminolevulinate-photodynamic therapy (PDT) with microneedling-assisted PDT on actinically damaged skin. Dermatol Surg. 2013;39(8):1197–201.

37. Harris AG, Naidoo C, Murrell DF. Skin needling as a treatment for acne scarring: an up-to-date review of the literature. Int J Womens Dermatol. 2015;1(2):77–81.

38. El-Domyati M, Barakat M, Awad S, Medhat W, El-Fakahany H, Farag H. Microneedling therapy for atrophic acne scars: an objective evaluation. J Clin Aesthet Dermatol. 2015;8(7):36–42.

39. Min S, Park SY, Yoon JY, Suh DH. Comparison of fractional microneedling radiofrequency and bipolar radiofrequency on acne and acne scar and investigation of mechanism: comparative randomized controlled clinical trial. Arch Dermatol Res. 2015;307(10):897–904.

40. Fabbrocini G, Marasca C, Ammad S, Brazzini B, Izzo R, Donnarumma M, et al. Assessment of the combined efficacy of needling and the use of silicone gel in the treatment of C-section and other surgical hypertrophic scars and keloids. Adv Skin Wound Care. 2016;29(9):408–11.

41. Mustoe TA. Evolution of silicone therapy and mechanism of action in scar management. Aesthetic Plast Surg. 2008;32(1):82–92.

42. Schwarz M, Laaff H. A prospective controlled assessment of microneedling with the Dermaroller device. Plast Reconstr Surg. 2011;127(6):146e–8e.

43. Majid I. Microneedling therapy in atrophic facial scars: an objective assessment. J Cutan Aesthet Surg. 2009;2(1):26–30.

44. Costa IM, Costa MC. Microneedling for varicella scars in a dark-skinned teenager. Dermatol Surg. 2014;40(3):333–4.

45. Park KY, Kim HK, Kim SE, Kim BJ, Kim MN. Treatment of striae distensae using needling therapy: a pilot study. Dermatol Surg. 2012;38(11):1823–8.

46. Aust MC, Knobloch K, Vogt PM. Percutaneous collagen induction therapy as a novel therapeutic option for Striae distensae. Plast Reconstr Surg. 2010;126(4):219e–20e.

47. Fabbrocini G, De Vita V, Fardella N, Pastore F, Annunziata MC, Mauriello MC, et al. Skin needling to enhance depigmenting serum penetration in the treatment of melasma. Plast Surg Int. 2011;2011:158241.

48. Lima Ede A. Microneedling in facial recalcitrant melasma: report of a series of 22 cases. An Bras Dermatol. 2015;90(6):919–21.

49. Sahni K, Kassir M. Dermafrac: an innovative new treatment for periorbital melanosis in a dark-skinned male patient. J Cutan Aesthet Surg. 2013;6(3):158–60.

50. Kontochristopoulos G, Kouris A, Platsidaki E, Markantoni V, Gerodimou M, Antoniou C. Combination of microneedling and 10% trichloroacetic acid peels in the management of infraorbital dark circles. J Cosmet Laser Ther. 2016;18(5):289–92.

51. Stanimirovic A, Kovacevic M, Korobko I, Situm M, Lotti T. Combined therapy for resistant vitiligo lesions: NB-UVB, microneedling, and topical latanoprost, showed no enhanced efficacy compared to topical latanoprost and NB-UVB. Dermatol Ther. 2016;29(5):312–6.

52. Mina M, Elgarhy L, Al-Saeid H, Ibrahim Z. Comparison between the efficacy of microneedling combined with 5-fluorouracil vs microneedling with tacrolimus in the treatment of vitiligo. J Cosmet Dermatol. 2018;17(5):744–51.

53. Dhurat R, Sukesh M, Avhad G, Dandale A, Pal A, Pund P. A randomized evaluator blinded study of effect of microneedling in androgenetic alopecia: a pilot study. Int J Trichology. 2013;5(1):6–11.

54. Dhurat R, Mathapati S. Response to microneedling treatment in men with androgenetic alopecia who failed to respond to conventional therapy. Indian J Dermatol. 2015;60(3):260–3.

55. Kwack MH, Sung YK, Chung EJ, Im SU, Ahn JS, Kim MK, et al. Dihydrotestosterone-inducible dickkopf 1 from balding dermal papilla cells causes apoptosis in follicular keratinocytes. J Invest Dermatol. 2008;128(2):262–9.

56. Kim YS, Jeong KH, Kim JE, Woo YJ, Kim BJ, Kang H. Repeated microneedle stimulation induces enhanced hair growth in a murine model. Ann Dermatol. 2016;28(5):586–92.

57. Jeong K, Lee Y, Kim J, Park Y, Kim B, Kang H. Repeated microneedle stimulation induce the enhanced expression of hair-growth-related genes. Int J Trichology. 2012;4:117.

58. Sharad J. Combination of microneedling and glycolic acid peels for the treatment of acne scars in dark skin. J Cosmet Dermatol. 2011;10(4):317–23.

59. Leheta TM, Abdel Hay RM, Hegazy RA, El Garem YF. Do combined alternating sessions of 1540 nm nonablative fractional laser and percutaneous collagen induction with trichloroacetic acid 20% show better results than each individual modality in the treatment of atrophic acne scars? A randomized controlled trial. J Dermatolog Treat. 2014;25(2):137–41.

60. Leheta TM, Abdel Hay RM, El Garem YF. Deep peeling using phenol versus percutaneous collagen induction combined with trichloroacetic acid 20% in atrophic post-acne scars; a randomized controlled trial. J Dermatolog Treat. 2014;25(2):130–6.

61. Hassan R. Comparison of efficacy of micro needling for the treatment of acne scars in Asian skin with and without subcision. J Turk Acad Dermatol. 2015;9(2):159–66.

62. Casabona G, Marchese P. Calcium hydroxylapatite combined with microneedling and ascorbic acid is effective for treating stretch marks. Plast Reconstr Surg Glob Open. 2017;5(9):e1474.

63. Hom DB, Linzie BM, Huang TC. The healing effects of autologous platelet gel on acute human skin wounds. Arch Facial Plast Surg. 2007;9(3):174–83.

64. Fabbrocini G, De Vita V, Pastore F, Panariello L. Combined use of skin needling and platelet-rich plasma in acne scarring treatment. Cosmet Dermatol. 2011;24(4):177–83.

65. Porwal S, Chahar YS, Singh PK. A comparative study of combined dermaroller and platelet-rich plasma versus dermaroller alone in acne scars and assessment of quality of life before and after treatment. Indian J Dermatol. 2018;63(5):403–8.

66. Nofal E, Helmy A, Nofal A, Alakad R, Nasr M. Platelet-rich plasma versus CROSS technique with 100% trichloroacetic acid versus combined skin needling and platelet rich plasma in the treatment of atrophic acne scars: a comparative study. Dermatol Surg. 2014;40(8):864–73.

67. Seo KY, Kim DH, Lee SE, Yoon MS, Lee HJ. Skin rejuvenation by microneedle fractional radiofrequency and a human stem cell conditioned medium in Asian skin: a randomized controlled investigator blinded split-face study. J Cosmet Laser Ther. 2013;15(1):25–33.

68. Kim WS, Park BS, Park SH, Kim HK, Sung JH. Antiwrinkle effect of adipose-derived stem cell: activation of dermal fibroblast by secretory factors. J Dermatol Sci. 2009;53(2):96–102.

69. Park BS, Jang KA, Sung JH, Park JS, Kwon YH, Kim KJ, et al. Adipose-derived stem cells and their secretory factors as a promising therapy for skin aging. Dermatol Surg. 2008;34(10):1323–6.

70. Lee MJ, Kim J, Lee KI, Shin JM, Chae JI, Chung HM. Enhancement of wound healing by secretory factors of endothelial precursor cells derived from human embryonic stem cells. Cytotherapy. 2011;13(2):165–78.

71. Cho SW, Moon SH, Lee SH, Kang SW, Kim J, Lim JM, et al. Improvement of postnatal neovascularization by human embryonic stem cell derived endothelial-like cell transplantation in a mouse model of hindlimb ischemia. Circulation. 2007;116(21):2409–19.

72. Chung JH, Youn SH, Kwon OS, Cho KH, Youn JI, Eun HC. Regulations of collagen synthesis by ascorbic acid, transforming growth factor-beta and interferon-gamma in human dermal fibroblasts cultured in three-dimensional collagen gel are photoaging- and aging-independent. J Dermatol Sci. 1997;15(3):188–200.

73. Lee HJ, Lee EG, Kang S, Sung JH, Chung HM, Kim DH. Efficacy of microneedling plus human stem cell conditioned medium for skin rejuvenation: a randomized, controlled, blinded split-face study. Ann Dermatol. 2014;26(5):584–91.

74. Fernandes D. Percutaneous collagen induction: an alternative to laser resurfacing. Aesthet Surg J. 2002;22(3):307–9.

75. Nusgens BV, Humbert P, Rougier A, Colige AC, Haftek M, Lambert CA, et al. Topically applied vitamin C enhances the mRNA level of collagens I and III, their processing enzymes and tissue inhibitor of matrix metalloproteinase 1 in the human dermis. J Invest Dermatol. 2001;116(6):853–9.

76. Kafi R, Kwak HS, Schumacher WE, Cho S, Hanft VN, Hamilton TA, et al. Improvement of naturally aged skin with vitamin A (retinol). Arch Dermatol. 2007;143(5):606–12.

77. Buchanan PJ, Gilman RH. Retinoids: Literature review and suggested algorithm for use prior to facial resurfacing procedures. J Cutan Aesthet Surg. 2016;9(3):139–44.

78. Glick AB, McCune BK, Abdulkarem N, Flanders KC, Lumadue JA, Smith JM, et al. Complex regulation of TGF beta expression by retinoic acid in the vitamin A-deficient rat. Development. 1991;111(4):1081–6.

79. Murad S, Grove D, Lindberg KA, Reynolds G, Sivarajah A, Pinnell SR. Regulation of collagen synthesis by ascorbic acid. Proc Natl Acad Sci U S A. 1981;78(5):2879–82.

80. Soltani-Arabshahi R, Wong JW, Duffy KL, Powell DL. Facial allergic granulomatous reaction and systemic hypersensitivity associated with microneedle therapy for skin rejuvenation. JAMA Dermatol. 2014;150(1):68–72.

81. Zahr AS, Kononov T, Sensing W, Biron JA, Gold MH. An open-label, single-site study to evaluate the tolerability, safety, and efficacy of using a novel facial moisturizer for preparation and accelerated healing pre and post a single full-face radiofrequency microneedling treatment. J Cosmet Dermatol. 2018; 18(1): 94–106.

82. Doddaballapur S. Microneedling with dermaroller. J Cutan Aesthet Surg. 2009;2(2):110–1.

83. Dogra S, Yadav S, Sarangal R. Microneedling for acne scars in Asian skin type: an effective low cost treatment modality. J Cosmet Dermatol. 2014;13(3):180–7.

84. Pahwa M, Pahwa P, Zaheer A. "Tram track effect" after treatment of acne scars using a microneedling device. Dermatol Surg. 2012;38(7 Pt 1):1107–8.
85. McCrudden MT, McAlister E, Courtenay AJ, Gonzalez-Vazquez P, Singh TR, Donnelly RF. Microneedle applications in improving skin appearance. Exp Dermatol. 2015;24(8):561–6.
86. Singh A, Yadav S. Microneedling: Advances and widening horizons. Indian Dermatol Online J. 2016;7(4):244–54.
87. Chandrashekar BS, Sriram R, Mysore R, Bhaskar S, Shetty A. Evaluation of microneedling fractional radiofrequency device for treatment of acne scars. J Cutan Aesthet Surg. 2014;7(2):93–7.
88. Vejjabhinanta V, Wanitphakdeedecha R, Limtanyakul P, Manuskiatti W. The efficacy in treatment of facial atrophic acne scars in Asians with a fractional radiofrequency microneedle system. J Eur Acad Dermatol Venereol. 2014;28(9):1219–25.
89. Cho SI, Chung BY, Choi MG, Baek JH, Cho HJ, Park CW, et al. Evaluation of the clinical efficacy of fractional radiofrequency microneedle treatment in acne scars and large facial pores. Dermatol Surg. 2012;38(7 Pt 1):1017–24.
90. Lee SJ, Goo JW, Shin J, Chung WS, Kang JM, Kim YK, et al. Use of fractionated microneedle radio-frequency for the treatment of inflammatory acne vulgaris in 18 Korean patients. Dermatol Surg. 2012;38(3):400–5.
91. Yadav S, Dogra S. A cutaneous reaction to microneedling for postacne scarring caused by nickel hyper-sensitivity. Aesthet Surg J. 2016;36(4):NP168–70.
92. Alster TS, Graham PM. Microneedling: a review and practical guide. Dermatol Surg. 2018;44(3):397–404.
93. Sasaki GH. Micro-needling depth penetration, presence of pigment particles, and fluorescein-stained platelets: clinical usage for aesthetic concerns. Aesthet Surg J. 2017;37(1):71–83.
94. Lima EVA, Lima MA, Takano D. Microneedling experimental study and classification of the resulting injury. Surgical and Cosmetic Dermatology. 2013;5(2):110–4.
95. Zeitter S, Sikora Z, Jahn S, Stahl F, Strauss S, Lazaridis A, et al. Microneedling: matching the results of medical needling and repetitive treatments to maximize potential for skin regeneration. Burns. 2014;40(5):966–73.

12

Dermatotoxicology of Microneedles in Man

John Havens Cary
Louisiana State University School of Medicine

Becky S. Li
Howard University College of Medicine

Howard I. Maibach
University of California, San Francisco, School of Medicine

The authors declare no conflict of interest.

12.1 Introduction

Microneedles (MNs), minimally invasive devices designed to painlessly penetrate the stratum corneum, were developed in 1976 as a means for more efficient transdermal drug delivery (Ma and Wu 2017). In subsequent decades, advancement in MN technology and manufacturing has led to development of several types of MNs including hollow, solid, dissolving, coated, and hydrogel-forming (Nguyen and Park 2018). Hollow MNs deliver drugs through a channel in a similar manner to hypodermic needles, while solid MNs are more frequently used in pretreatment to enhance the permeability of the skin before application of a topical product. Dissolving MNs are constructed from a biodegradable polymer or polysaccharide with therapeutic molecules contained within; coated MNs contain the drug formulation on the outside surface of the needles. Lastly, hydrogel-forming MNs are made of expanding material with an active agent attached to the baseplate (Nguyen and Park 2018). Current and potential applications of MNs include: dermal and intrascleral drug delivery, vaccine administration, blood and interstitial fluid extraction, and numerous uses in cosmetics (Ramaut et al. 2018; Ma and Wu 2017).

The MNs allow delivery of higher-molecular-weight and hydrophilic drugs that would otherwise be unable to diffuse across the stratum corneum. In contrast to enteral drug delivery, dermal drug delivery avoids stomach degradation and hepatic first-pass metabolism, while it may also produce higher drug concentrations in the dermis and other target tissues. Badran et al. (2009) demonstrated effective penetration of radiolabeled mannitol, a hydrophilic drug expected to have poor penetration into the stratum corneum, in full-thickness human skin grafts when combined with microneedling. Dhurat et al. found enhanced effectiveness of minoxidil in men with androgenetic alopecia when used in conjunction with micronneedling in comparison to conventional minoxidil treatment; they also demonstrated effectiveness of MN and minoxidil combination therapy in patients who failed to respond to conventional minoxidil treatment (Dhurat et al. 2013; Dhurat and Mathapati 2015). Jiang et al. (2009) demonstrated effective intrascleral delivery of microparticles via MNs. With possible drug diffusion to surrounding tissues like the choroid, retina, and ciliary body, intrascleral drug delivery via MNs has the potential to treat posterior eye disease such as glaucoma and macular degeneration, although further research is needed (Jiang et al. 2009).

The MN delivery of vaccines releases antigenic material into the viable dermis, which has shown stronger immunological reactions when compared to muscle, the delivery target of traditional hypodermic needles (Engelke et al. 2015). A multi-center, randomized open-label study of 978 healthy adults showed intradermal influenza vaccine delivered by microinjection systems to convey a non-inferior humoral response against three influenza strains and two superior humoral responses to both A strains (H1N1, H3N2) (Leroux-Roels et al. 2008). Similar studies on influenza vaccination have demonstrated comparable or superior responses when compared to responses from conventional intramuscular vaccination

(Van Damme et al. 2009; Kenney et al. 2004). In addition to potentially less expensive and superior humoral responses for some vaccines, MNs eliminate sharp, bio-hazardous waste and painful injections present in vaccines administered via hypodermic needles.

Development of optimized hollow MNs has resulted in additional potential applications, including blood and interstitial fluid extraction (Li et al. 2013; Kiang et al. 2017). When paired with biosensors and other microsystems, MNs have the potential for use in glucose and drug monitoring (Kiang et al. 2017). While experiments with MN-integrated biosensors have yielded promising results, extensive preclinical and clinical trials are needed before their implementation as point-of-care devices for ISF collection, drug concentration assessment, or dosing in real time (Kiang et al. 2017).

Dermal microneedling has proven an effective therapy for atrophic acne scars and skin rejuvenation (Kim et al. 2011). Although the exact mechanism is unknown, MN puncture likely disrupts older collagen strands and promotes damaged collagen removal (Fabbrocini et al. 2009). In addition, rolling with multiple MNs to promote new collagen and elastin deposition, known as collagen induction therapy, has become popular practice in treating disfiguring scars and rhytides and rejuvenating skin (Fabbrocini et al. 2009; Aust et al. 2008). Other methods used to improve the clinical appearance of acne scarring such as laser resurfacing carry risks associated with a disrupted skin epidermal barrier. Cho et al. (2012) showed microneedling to lead to improved grade of acne scars and global assessment of large pores in more than 70% of 30 tested patients. Kim et al. (2011) compared the effects of microneedling to those of intense pulsed light therapy for skin rejuvenation, finding significantly higher levels of collagen in microneedling when evaluated via caliper, microscopic examination, Western blot analysis for type I collagen, and enzyme-linked immunosorbent assay for total collagen content.

12.2 Adverse Events

Perhaps the most extensive use of MNs in any one application occurs with collagen-induction therapy. Consequently, most discussion of adverse events and normal post-procedural expectations involve this application.

Common contraindications to MN collagen-induction therapy include active acne; herpes labialis or other active current infection such as impetigo or warts; patients on anticoagulant therapy such as warfarin and heparin or with other blood dyscrasias; patients with extreme keloid scarring tendency; and patients on chemotherapy, radiotherapy, or high doses of corticosteroids (Singh and Yadav 2016; Fernandes 2005).

In the healthy patient without contraindication to treatment, typical post-procedural expectations in collagen induction therapy with MNs include bleeding, bruising, erythema, and irritation (Fernandes 2005). Fernandes (2005) outlines a predicted appearance timeline and general recommendations following percutaneous collagen induction. Patients may note a bruised skin appearance with a swollen face following collagen induction therapy with a minimal, temporary ooze of serum. He recommends soaking the skin with saline swabs for 1–2 hours followed by treatment with a tea-tree-oil cleanser, while also encouraging patients to use topical vitamin A and vitamin C cream or oil to enhance healing. However, it is important that patients use only topical products approved for intradermal use, as inappropriate topical formula in conjunction with MN therapy increases the potential for allergic and irritant reactions. Note that vitamin A is known to aggravate flush and cause dry, flaky skin. Patients should thoroughly wash their face until all serum, blood, and oil is removed to prevent any minor eschar formation, as minor eschars may result in development of simple milia or tiny pustules. The skin should look less dramatic following day 1 with moderate flush on day 4 to 5 and very few visible signs post-procedure day 7. Patients should avoid unapproved topical formulations for at least 24 hours and refrain from direct sun exposure for at least 10 days. Fernandes advises at least 1 month in between retreatment with MNs, although the optimal interval is not currently known.

Despite the potential uses and existence for over 4 decades, MNs have yet to be fully integrated into the medical system. The following discussion investigates potential side effects of MNs, including infection, irritation and irritant contact dermatitis (ICD), allergic contact dermatitis (ACD), hyperpigmentation, abnormal scarring, and irritant and allergic granulomas. We also consider the potential for photoirritation/phototoxicity, photoallergic contact dermatitis, non-immunologic contact urticaria, and immunologic contact urticaria. For a summary of literature documenting adverse events with MNs, please see Table 12.1.

12.2.1 Infection

The stratum corneum serves many purposes, including a physical defense against microorganisms. Microchannels formed during MN therapy have the potential to facilitate access of microorganisms and increase susceptibility to infection. Gupta et al. (2011) evaluated the kinetics of stratum corneum

TABLE 12.1

Literature Documenting Adverse Events to MNs

Adverse Reaction Type	Author(s) and Year	Number of Patients	Additional Details
Infection	Aust et al. (2008)	2	2/480 patients with herpes simplex infection
	Torezan et al. (2013)	1	1/10 patients with infection based on symptoms
	Cunha et al. (2017)	1	*Microsporum canis* infection of bilateral arms and legs
ICD	Cercal Fucci-da-Costa and Reich Camasmie (2018)	1	Suspected irritation to arnica-based cream
ACD	Yadav and Dogra (2016)	1	"Rail track appearance" of adverse reaction with positive patch test to nickel
Allergic/irritant granulomas[1]	Soltani-Arabshahi et al. (2014)	3	Two patients with granulomatous reaction, systemic symptoms, and +1 reaction to Vita C serum; one patient with granulomatous reaction and no systemic symptoms
Irregular scarring	Pahwa et al. (2012)[2]	1	"Tram tracking" appearance over temporal area, zygomatic arch, and forehead
	Dogra et al. (2014)[2]	2	2/36 patients in study with a "tram track" adverse event; 1/2 "tram trek" patients withdrawn from study
Post-inflammatory hyperpigmentation	Dogra et al. (2014)	5	5/36 patients in study; 3/5 patients forced to withdraw from study; 2/5 patients improved with photoprotection
	Sharad (2011)	4	4/36 patients in study with more transient hyperpigmentation
	Majid (2009)	1	1/37 patients in study with transient hyperpigmentation

[1] Allergic/irritant granulomas may be considered a subset of ICD or ACD.

[2] "Tram tracking" or "tram trek" lesions may be due to ICD or ACD, as the authors did not determine the underlying cause.

resealing in MN versus hypodermic needles, finding faster resealing in MN-treated skin. Donnelly et al. (2009) evaluated the microbial penetration in hypodermic needles versus MN-induced holes in Silescol® membranes and neonate porcine skin. They demonstrated significantly lower penetration of *Candida albicans, Pseudomonas aeruguinosa*, and *Staphylococcus epidermidis* across viable epidermis in MN than with hypodermic needle puncture. Vicente-Perez et al. (2017) evaluated the effect of MN patches on mice, testing for biomarkers of inflammation and infection, weight, and several other variables. They found no detectable levels of TNF-α among mice and no statistically significant increase in C-reactive protein, immunoglobulin G, or interleukin 1-beta in MN-tested mice in comparison to control mice, regardless of formulation type, needle density, number of applications, or mouse sex ($p > 0.05$ in all cases). In addition, mice in all study and control groups demonstrated increased weight over the course of the study. Collectively, the authors were unable to detect any infection or any variable indicative of an infection across all tested mice.

Aust et al. (2008) performed a retrospective analysis of 480 patients with fine wrinkles, lax skin, scarring, and striae gravidarum treated with percutaneous collagen induction using the Medical Roll-CIT with topical vitamins A and C cosmetic creams for a minimum of 4 weeks postoperatively. Two patients developed herpes simplex infection following a full-face needling that was successfully treated with acyclovir.

In a pilot split-face study comparing conventional methyl aminolevulinate-photodynamic therapy (PDT) with microneedling-assisted PDT on actinically damaged skin, 1 of 10 patients developed an infection on the MN-treated side 7 days post-treatment, determined by signs and symptoms of high local temperature, redness, pain, and crusts (Torezan et al. 2013).

Cunha et al. (2017) document a case of tinea corporis that emerged in corresponding locations of dermaroller use approximately 3 weeks after start of her home MN therapy for bilateral scarring of her arms and legs. Potassium hydroxide examination of the lesions was positive for fungus with lesion culture growing *Microsporum canis*. While the patient confirmed skin-cleaning prior and sanitation of the MN device before and after therapy, inadequate sterilization of the patient's skin and MN device cannot be excluded.

Leatham et al. (2018) document a case of facial autoinoculation of varicella via a home microneedling roller device. A healthy woman with a distant history of primary varicella zoster virus (VZV) infection and no prior shingles vaccination reported grouped lesions over her chest, which she presumed an acneiform eruption. The patient self-treated the area with an at-home microneedling roller device and used the device over her face to reduce the appearance of rhytides. On presentation, the patient had "grouped, eroded papules and vesicles on the right T4 dermatome" and "eroded papules on the forehead, lateral cheeks, many located at spaced distances." PCR yielded positive results for VZV. Patient was started on oral valacyclovir and was free of lesions and experienced no postherpetic neuralgia at 6 weeks.

12.2.2 Irritant Contact Dermatitis

The ICD is an eczematous-like reaction occurring from contact with a chemical, biological, or physical agent (Tan et al. 2014). Severity of the reaction is dependent upon the physiochemical property of the agent and the degree of activation of the innate immune system (Tan et al. 2014). Keratinocytes, which comprise 95% of epidermal cells, are responsible for production of the majority of cytokines likely responsible for the ensuing erythema and edema (Tan et al. 2014). In contact with any agent, there is potential for ICD; however, it is likely that disruption of the stratum corneum provides increased susceptibility to a particular irritant. MNs are most frequently manufactured from non-irritating metal, polymer, silicon, and glass, none of which are particularly common irritants (Nguyen and Park 2018). However, irritation following a procedure may result from the MNs themselves or any substance used in conjunction.

Cercal Fucci-da-Costa and Reich Camasmie (2018) document a case of likely ICD due to skin rejuvenation MN therapy over the patient's dorsal hands. Following her MN therapy, the patient inadvertently applied arnica-based cream and developed yellowish papules compatible with MN perforation sites on an erythematous base 48 hours post-arnica cream application. The authors attributed the lesions to ICD from the arnica-based cream due to the sparing of MN-treated areas in which the cream was not applied and the patient's improvement 72 hours post–topical corticosteroid treatment.

Soltani-Arabshahi et al. (2014) document three cases of post-MN therapy granulomatous presentation of possible irritant or allergic origin discussed in "Allergic/Irritant Granulomas." In addition, it is likely that MN-related ICD is significantly underreported in the literature. Assessment of post-procedural erythema allows a rough estimate of the irritation incurred during the procedure. However, post-procedural erythema is likely dependent on factors such as: MN application site, amount of MN applications, MN length and type, combination therapy with topical products, and variability between skin types.

Bal et al. (2008) applied MN arrays (200, 300, or 400 µm solid metal MN arrays and 300 or 550 µm hollow metal MN arrays) using a standardized electrical applicator to the forearms of 18 human volunteers and measured redness using skin color assessment and laser Doppler imaging. They found longer needle lengths to result in greater irritation, evidenced by the 400 µm solid MNs resulting in significantly greater change in redness in comparison to the 200 µm solid MNs ($P < 0.001$). Lastly, they concluded 15 minutes post-application as the maximum change in redness with minimal irritation lasting less than 2 hours for all MNs.

Gill et al. (2008) investigated safety of single, longer MN lengths (480, 700, 960, and 1450 µm) on the volar forearm of healthy human volunteers, finding decreasing erythema over 2 hours in all subjects with no excessive erythema self-reported by research subjects when contacted at 24 hours.

Han et al. (2012) used a chromameter to measure post-treatment erythema following MN therapy using 150 and 250 µm MN rollers over one side of the face of healthy human volunteers. They found recovery time to baseline erythema to be 24 hours in the 5-application group and 48 hours in the 10-application group and a significant difference in the erythema index ratio between the two groups after 24 hours ($p = 0.002$). In contrast, they did not find a significant difference between the erythema index ratio of the 150 and 200 µm MN roller groups, although the mean erythema index ratios were higher in the 250 µm MN roller group.

12.2.3 Allergic Contact Dermatitis

The ACD is a type IV hypersensitivity reaction requiring prior sensitization and re-exposure to the allergen (Mowad et al. 2016). In the sensitization phase, the unprocessed chemical allergen, known as a hapten, penetrates the lower levels of the epidermis, where it is engulfed by a Langerhans cell and later presented to T-cells (Marks and deLeo 2016). Upon subsequent exposure to the allergen, cell-mediated immune response results in an eczematous-like lesion. As previously mentioned, microneedling disrupts the stratum corneum, increasing the ability of molecules, possibly allergens, to enter the dermis.

Yadav and Dogra (2016) identified a potential case of ACD occurring as a result of a microneedling procedure for the treatment of atrophic acne facial scars. Other than a local anesthetic applied 1 hour before and completely cleaned with normal saline and betadine, no serum or chemical was applied before, during, or after the procedure. The patient developed erythema and edema over the next 2 days, which gradually subsided. Simultaneously, the patient developed vesiculopustular lesions and erythematous papules arranged linearly along the lines of the microneedling device, giving a "rail track appearance." The lesions cleared in 4 weeks, and after 3 months, she was patch-tested with both nickel sulfate (5% in petroleum) and titanium (10% in petroleum) with readings taken at 48 and 96 hours. The patient demonstrated a negative reaction to titanium patch testing and experienced tiny vesiculopustular lesions and intense erythema, extending beyond the margins at 48 hours in response to nickel.

Of note is that Pahwa et al. (2012) and Dogra et al. (2014) document cases of "tram tracking" and "tram trek" scarring respectively. It is unclear whether Yadav and Dogra's documentation of a "rail track"-appearing reaction represents a similar or a distinct entity. However, the former authors were unable to attribute the scarring to a particular allergen or irritant, so they are discussed here in section 12.2.5 below.

12.2.4 Allergic/Irritant Chronic Inflammatory Reactions and Granulomas

Granulomatous inflammation is most commonly characterized by a collection of histiocytes (macrophages) surrounding an antigenic center, which may occasionally be necrotic; however, granulomatous inflammation encompasses presentations ranging from a well-organized granuloma to loose aggregates of epithelioid cells mixed with other inflammatory cells (Shah et al. 2017). Granulomas may develop with or without immunologic modulation in the case of granulomatous hypersensitivity and foreign-body granulomas respectively (Epstein 1989). Dermal granulomatous hypersensitivity has historically been associated with intradermal tattooing of red dyes with metallic elements and injection of dermal fillers such as hyaluronic acid and poly-L-lactic acid (PLA).

Pratsou and Gach (2013) report two sisters who underwent a facial microneedling procedure with a trained practitioner using a CE-marked,[1] US Food and Drug Administration (FDA)-registered device coupled with skin cleansing and topical anesthetic cream. Within 24 hours, both sisters developed significant lymphadenopathy, and the older sister developed pinpoint erythema, malaise, and headache. Systemic antibiotics were unhelpful, as the older sister's condition worsened with a "florid erythematous papular rash over her face" with spread to her trunk and limbs. The patient gradually improved over 2 weeks with systemic and topical corticosteroid treatment. Biopsy of lesions showed a nonspecific, chronic inflammatory infiltrate. Patch testing yielded a positive reaction to nickel sulfate (D4++), a known allergy to the patient. The authors were unable to attribute the reaction to her allergy, as the MN device contained up to 0.006% sulfur and 8% nickel bound to surgical-grade stainless steel (per manufacturer)—an amount thought to pose little or no risk in short-term contact with nickel-sensitive individuals.

Soltani-Arabshahi et al. (2014) document a total of three cases of granulomatous reactions to MN therapy. In the first case, two women presented after Dermapen MN therapy followed by high dose of lipophilic vitamin C (Vita C Serum; Sanítas Skincare) applied to the skin at the same medical spa. Both patients developed a progressive erythematous rash over the face in addition to systemic reactions, including arthralgias of varying intensity. In both cases, biopsy of indurated papules showed foreign-body-type granulomatous reaction with focal, polarizable material present in giant cell cytoplasm. Patch testing both patients showed +1 reaction to Vita C Serum, while patch testing with Vita C Serum in five healthy volunteers yielded negative reactions. Both patients had persistent, mildly indurated, erythematous papules and plaques at 9-month follow-up. In the last of the three cases, patients presented following three microneedling procedures, two in which a gel product (Boske Hydra-Boost Gel; Boske Dermaceuticals) and one in which Vital Pigment Stabilizer (Dermapen, LLC) were applied before microneedling. In the last of the three cases, patients underwent three consecutive microneedling procedures, two in which a gel product (Boske Hydra-Boost Gel; Boske Dermaceuticals) and one in which Vital Pigment Stabilizer (Dermapen, LLC) were applied before microneedling. While none of the patients experienced systemic symptoms in any of the procedures, one presented with a progressively worsening erythematous rash that developed papular features, with biopsy showing a similar granulomatous reaction. However, she refused patch testing and demonstrated resolution at 3 weeks.

12.2.5 Irregular Scarring

Pahwa et al. (2012) reported "tram tracking" or multiple discrete papular scars in a linear pattern in the horizontal and vertical directions in a 25-year-old woman 1 month after treatment with a dermal rolling device for management of post-acne scarring. The scarring was predominantly located over the temporal area, zygomatic arch, and the forehead of the patient, who slightly improved with topical silicone gel at 6-month follow-up. They were unable to attribute the atypical scarring to an allergen or irritant.

Dogra et al. (2014) reported 2/36 patients undergoing MN therapy for atrophic acne scars to have a similar "tram trek" adverse effect. One patient developed severe tram trek scarring over the malar prominence and was forced to withdraw; however, the patient did improve with topical tretinoin. The second patient developed less severe tram trek scarring over the forehead and was able to complete the study.

It is possible that the "tram trek" scarring may be a result of excessive force during the microneedling procedure over bony prominences of the patient's face.

12.2.6 Post-Inflammatory Hyperpigmentation

Post-inflammatory hyperpigmentation (PIH) is a hypermelanosis resulting from dermal inflammation or injury most commonly in people with skin of color (Davis and Callender 2010). The inflammation may be endogenous in the case of primary dermatoses or exogenous from external insults such

---

[1] The CE mark indicates that the manufacturer of a product takes responsibility for the compliance of this product with all applicable European health, safety, performance and environmental requirements.

as trauma or physical injury (Epstein 1989). While the pathogenesis is not completely known, PIH is believed to result from increased production of melanin or increased release of melanin due to melanocyte-stimulating signals such as cytokines and various other inflammatory mediators (Davis and Callender 2010).

Dogra et al. (2014) found 5/36 patients to present with PIH following 2–3 treatments of MN therapy for post-acne scarring. Of the five patients, three had severe hyperpigmentation forcing them to withdraw from the study, while the other two gradually improved with photoprotection.

Sharad (2011) and Majid (2009) reported more transient PIH in 4/36 patients and 1/37 patients respectively in similar studies on MN therapy for atrophic scarring. Each of the previously mentioned cases of hyperpigmentation featured phototype III or greater skin, except for one patient of unspecified type. To date, the amount of adverse hyperpigmentation reactions remains minimal and is possibly a result of improper UV protection following the procedure (Ramaut et al. 2018).

12.2.7 Other Adverse Effects to Consider

Lastly, other reactions of which MN users should be aware are photoirritation, photoallergy, non-immunologic contact urticaria (NICU), and mmunologic contact urticaria (ICU).

Phototoxic, or photoirritant, reactions are evoked from the combination of an exogenous or endogenous compound and ultraviolet (UV) irradiation (Ibbotson 2014). Phototoxic reactions most often appear similar to an acute sunburn; however, they occasionally present with urticarial, eczematous, lichenoid, or, rarely, pigmentary changes (Maibach and Honari 2014). In contrast, photoallergy requires a prior sensitization to the chemical in the presence of UV radiation and an additional exposure, in which there is a cell-mediated immune response and clinical presentation of the photoallergy (Ibbotson 2014). Photoallergic reactions most often present with eczematous-like changes (Maibach and Honari 2014).

Contact urticaria comprises a group of inflammatory reactions ranging from itching, burning, and tingling to systemic anaphylaxis (Gimenez-Arnau and Maibach 2014). Contact urticaria can be divided into NICU and ICU, the two separate entities being distinguished by immunologic memory in the case of ICU but no required prior sensitization in NICU (Gimenez-Arnau and Maibach 2014). The ICU and NICU are distinct in mechanism and etiology, but have very subtle, if any, difference in their clinical presentation (Gimenez-Arnau and Maibach 2014; Lahti 2000).

There is little to no current literature documenting photoirritation, photoallergy, NICU, or ICU resulting from MN therapy; however, we believe they are conditions of which it is important to be aware in view of the potential growth of MN use in the future.

12.3 Conclusion

Of all MN applications, the growth of MN use in the cosmetics industry for skin rejuvenation in the spa or the home setting raises the most concern. As previously mentioned, skin rejuvenation with MNs or collagen-induction therapy represents the most extensive use of MNs in any one therapy of all potential MN applications. In addition, skin rejuvenation is frequently performed outside of the medical setting, which also increases the chance of adverse events, especially those stemming from improper sterilization or the coupling inappropriate topical products. We advise patients to understand contraindications for use and follow post-therapy guidelines, especially when seeking therapy outside of the medical setting.

Ramaut et al. (2018) systematically reviewed the MN literature and its potential application in atrophic acne scars, skin rejuvenation, hypertrophic scars, keloids, striae distensae, androgenetic alopecia, melasma, and acne vulgaris. They generally favored MN therapy due to minimal side effects with shorter recovery periods and similar results when compared to other treatments.

In addition, various clinical trials involving MNs that are completed, active, or recruiting are listed in Table 12.2. Some of the more common clinical trial applications include uveitis with five and actinic keratosis with three clinical trials completed, ongoing, or recruiting.

TABLE 12.2

Completed, Active, and Recruiting Clinical Trials Involving MNs in the United States According to ClinicalTrials.gov*

Clinical Trial Course	Targeted Application	Number of Trials	Trial Phase	Enrollment (Number of Patients)	Age of Patients (Years)
Completed	Type I diabetes	1	2, 3	16	8–18
	Hyperhydrosis	1	1	13	12+
	Actinic keratosis	3	N/A; N/A; 2	33; 51; 137	18+
	Intracutaneous drug delivery	1	N/A	12	18–49
	Uveitis	4	1; 2; 3; 3; 2	11; 38; 160; 22	18+
	Overactive bladder	1	N/A	8	18+
	Acute migraine	1	2, 3	365	18–65
	Atopic dermatitis	2	1; N/A	40; 368	18–64
	Postmenopausal osteoporosis	2	1; 2	24; 250	55–85; up to 85
	Polio immunity	1	2	231	18–90
	Diabetic macular edema	1	1, 2	20	18+
	Influenza	1	N/A	24	18–49
Active	Influenza	1	1	100	18–49
	Type I diabetes	1	2	20	18+
	Face and neck wrinkles, texture, pigmentation	1	N/A	21	18+
	Diabetic macular edema	1	2	71	18+
Recruiting	Macular edema, retinal vein occlusion	1	3	460	18+
	Vaccination, skin absorption	1	N/A	50	6 weeks–24 months
	Diabetes	1	N/A	15	7–18
	Wrinkles	1	N/A	32	22+
	Cutaneous T-cell lymphoma	1	1	54	18+
	Skin laxity	1	N/A	20	18–75
	Migraine	1	3	250	18–75
	Uveitis	1	3	38	18+

* Note that there are two additional trials testing MN systems in healthy patients.

We believe MNs may be a relatively safe alternative and, in some circumstances, a superior option to many conventional therapies. However, further research and experience is needed to clarify the most appropriate and safe way to utilize this technology.

REFERENCES

Aust MC, Fernandes D, Kolokythas P, Kaplan HM, Vogt PM. Percutaneous Collagen Induction Therapy: An Alternative Treatment for Scars, Wrinkles, and Skin Laxity. Plastic and Reconstructive Surgery. 2008;121(4):1421–9. doi:10.1097/01.prs.0000304612.72899.02

Badran MM, Kuntsche J, Fahr A. Skin Penetration Enhancement by a Microneedle Device (Dermaroller®) In Vitro: Dependency on Needle Size and Applied Formulation. European Journal of Pharmaceutical Sciences. 2009;36(4):511–23. doi:https://doi.org/10.1016/j.ejps.2008.12.008

Bal SM, Caussin J, Pavel S, Bouwstra JA. In Vivo Assessment of Safety of Microneedle Arrays in Human Skin. European Journal of Pharmaceutical Sciences. 2008;35(3):193–202. doi:https://doi.org/10.1016/j.ejps.2008.06.016

Bariya SH, Gohel MC, Mehta TA, Sharma OP. Microneedles: An Emerging Transdermal Drug Delivery System. Journal of Pharmacy and Pharmacology. 2012;64(1):11–29.doi:10.1111/j.2042-7158.2011.01369.x

Cercal Fucci-da-Costa AP, Reich Camasmie H. Drug Delivery after Microneedling: Report of an Adverse Reaction. Dermatologic Surgery. 2018;44(4):593–4. doi:10.1097/dss.0000000000001250

Cho SI, Chung BY, Choi MG, Baek JH, Cho HJ, Park CW et al. Evaluation of the Clinical Efficacy of Fractional Radiofrequency Microneedle Treatment in Acne Scars and Large Facial Pores. Dermatologic Surgery. 2012;38(7pt1):1017–24. doi:10.1111/j.1524-4725.2012.02402.x

Cunha NMMd, Campos SLdA, Fidalgo AIPC. Unusual Presentation of Tinea Corporis Associated with the Use of a Microneedling Device. Aesthetic Surgery Journal. 2017;37(7):NP69–NP72. doi:10.1093/asj/sjx086

Davis EC, Callender VD. Postinflammatory Hyperpigmentation: A Review of the Epidemiology, Clinical Features, and Treatment Options in Skin of Color. The Journal of Clinical and Aesthetic Dermatology. 2010;3(7):20–31.

Dhurat R, Mathapati S. Response to Microneedling Treatment in Men With Androgenetic Alopecia Who Failed to Respond to Conventional Therapy. Indian Journal of Dermatology. 2015;60(3):260–3. doi:10.4103/0019-5154.156361

Dhurat R, Sukesh M, Avhad G, Dandale A, Pal A, Pund P. A Randomized Evaluator Blinded Study of Effect of Microneedling in Androgenetic Alopecia: A Pilot Study. International Journal of Trichology. 2013;5(1):6–11. doi:10.4103/0974-7753.114700

Dogra S, Yadav S, Sarangal R. Microneedling for Acne Scars in Asian Skin Type: An Effective Low Cost Treatment Modality. Journal of Cosmetic Dermatology. 2014;13(3):180–7.doi:10.1111/jocd.12095

Donnelly RF, Singh TRR, Tunney MM, Morrow DIJ, McCarron PA, O'Mahony C et al. Microneedle Arrays Allow Lower Microbial Penetration Than Hypodermic Needles In Vitro. Pharmaceutical Research. 2009;26(11):2513–22. doi:10.1007/s11095-009-9967-2

Engelke L, Winter G, Hook S, Engert J. Recent Insights into Cutaneous Immunization: How to Vaccinate Via the Skin. Vaccine. 2015;33(37):4663–74. doi:https://doi.org/10.1016/j.vaccine.2015.05.012

Epstein JH. Postinflammatory Hyperpigmentation. Clinics in Dermatology. 1989;7(2):55–65. doi:10.1016/0738-081X(89)90057-6

Epstein WL, Fukuyama K. Mechanisms of Granulomatous Inflammation. Immunol Ser. 1989;46:687–721.

Fabbrocini G, Fardella N, Monfrecola A, Proietti I,Innocenzi D. Acne Scarring Treatment Using Skin Needling. Clinical and Experimental Dermatology. 2009;34(8):874–9. doi:10.1111/j.1365-2230.2009.03291.x

Fernandes D. Minimally invasive percutaneous collagen induction. Oral. Maxillofac. Surg. Clin. 17(1), 51-63 (2005).

Gill HS, Denson DD, Burris BA, Prausnitz MR. Effect of Microneedle Design on Pain in Human Subjects. The Clinical Journal of Pain. 2008;24(7):585–94. doi:10.1097/AJP.0b013e31816778f9

Gimenez-Arnau AM, Maibach HI. Contact Urticaria Syndrome. CRC Press; 2014.

Gupta J, Gill HS, Andrews SN, Prausnitz MR. Kinetics of Skin Resealing after Insertion of Microneedles in Human Subjects. Journal of Controlled Release. 2011;154(2):148–55. doi:https://doi.org/10.1016/j.jconrel.2011.05.021

Ibbotson SH. Chapter 5—Photoallergic Contact Dermatitis: Clinical Aspects A2—Maibach, Howard. In: Honari G, editor. Applied Dermatotoxicology. Boston: Academic Press; 2014. p. 85–114.

Jiang J, Moore JS, Edelhauser HF, Prausnitz MR. Intrascleral Drug Delivery to the Eye Using Hollow Microneedles. Pharmaceutical Research. 2009;26(2):395–403. doi:10.1007/s11095-008-9756-3

Kenney RT, Frech SA, Muenz LR, Villar CP, Glenn GM. Dose Sparing with Intradermal Injection of Influenza Vaccine. New England Journal of Medicine. 2004;351(22):2295–301. doi:10.1056/NEJMoa043540

Kiang T, Ranamukhaarachchi S, Ensom M. Revolutionizing Therapeutic Drug Monitoring with the Use of Interstitial Fluid and Microneedles Technology. Pharmaceutics. 2017;9(4):43.

Kim SE, Lee JH, Kwon HB, Ahn BJ, Lee AY. Greater Collagen Deposition with the Microneedle Therapy System than with Intense Pulsed Light. Dermatologic Surgery. 2011;37(3):336–41. doi:10.1111/j.1524-4725.2011.01882.x

Lahti A. Non-Immunologic Contact Urticaria. In: Kanerva L, Wahlberg JE, Elsner P, Maibach HI, editors. Handbook of Occupational Dermatology. Berlin, Heidelberg: Springer Berlin Heidelberg; 2000. p. 221–4.

Leatham H, Guan L, Chang ALS. Unintended Widespread Facial Autoinoculation of Varicella by Home Microneedling Roller Device. JAAD Case Reports. 2018;4(6):546–7. doi:https://doi.org/10.1016/j.jdcr.2018.02.004

Leroux-Roels I, Vets E, Freese R, Seiberling M, Weber F, Salamand C et al. Seasonal Influenza Vaccine Delivered by Intradermal Microinjection: A Randomised Controlled Safety and Immunogenicity Trial in Adults. Vaccine. 2008;26(51):6614–9. doi:https://doi.org/10.1016/j.vaccine.2008.09.078

Li CG, Lee CY, Lee K, Jung H. An Optimized Hollow Microneedle for Minimally Invasive Blood Extraction. Biomedical Microdevices. 2013;15(1):17–25. doi:10.1007/s10544-012-9683-2

Lowe NJ, Maxwell CA, Patnaik R. Adverse Reactions to Dermal Fillers: Review. Dermatologic Surgery. 2005;31(s4):1626–33. doi:doi:10.2310/6350.2005.31250

Ma G, Wu C. Microneedle, Bio-microneedle and Bio-inspired Microneedle: A Review. Journal of Controlled Release. 2017;251:11–23. doi:https://doi.org/10.1016/j.jconrel.2017.02.011

Maibach H, Honari G. Chapter 3—Photoirritation (Phototoxicity): Clinical Aspects. In: Applied Dermatotoxicology. Boston: Academic Press; 2014. p. 41–56.

Majid I. Microneedling Therapy in Atrophic Facial Scars: An Objective Assessment. Journal of Cutaneous and Aesthetic Surgery. 2009;2(1):26–30. doi:10.4103/0974-2077.53096

Mang R, Stege H, Krutmann J. Mechanisms of Phototoxic and Photoallergic Reactions. In: Johansen JD, Frosch PJ, Lepoittevin JP, editors. Contact Dermatitis. Berlin, Heidelberg: Springer Berlin Heidelberg; 2011. p. 155–63.

Marks JG, DeLeo VA. Contact & Occupational Dermatology. Jaypee Brothers, Medical Publishers Pvt. Limited; 2016.

Mowad CM, Anderson B, Scheinman P, Pootongkam S, Nedorost S, Brod B. Allergic Contact Dermatitis: Patient Management and Education. Journal of the American Academy of Dermatology. 2016;74(6):1043–54. doi:https://doi.org/10.1016/j.jaad.2015.02.1144

Nguyen TT, Park JH. Human studies with microneedles for evaluation of their efficacy and safety. Expert. Opin. Drug. Deliv. 15(3), 235–45 (2018).

Pahwa M, Pahwa P, Zaheer A. "Tram Track Effect" after Treatment of Acne Scars Using a Microneedling Device. Dermatologic Surgery. 2012;38(7):1107–8. doi:10.1111/j.1524-4725.2012.02441.x

Pratsou P, Gach J. Severe Systemic Reaction Associated with Skin Microneedling Therapy in 2 Sisters: A Previously Unrecognized Potential for Complications? J Am Acad Dermatol. 2013;68(4):6447.

Ramaut L, Hoeksema H, Pirayesh A, Stillaert F, Monstrey S. Microneedling: Where Do We Stand Now? A Systematic Review of the Literature. Journal of Plastic, Reconstructive & Aesthetic Surgery. 2018;71(1):1–14. doi:10.1016/j.bjps.2017.06.006

Shah KK, Pritt BS, Alexander MP. Histopathologic Review of Granulomatous Inflammation. Journal of Clinical Tuberculosis and Other Mycobacterial Diseases. 2017;7:1–12. doi:https://doi.org/10.1016/j.jctube.2017.02.001

Sharad J. Combination of Microneedling and Glycolic Acid Peels for the Treatment of Acne Scars in Dark Skin. Journal of Cosmetic Dermatology. 2011;10(4):317–23. doi:doi:10.1111/j.1473-2165.2011.00583.x

Singh A, Yadav S. Microneedling: Advances and Widening Horizons. Indian Dermatology Online Journal. 2016;7(4):244–54. doi:10.4103/2229-5178.185468

Soltani-Arabshahi R, Wong JW, Duffy KL, Powell DL. Facial Allergic Granulomatous Reaction and Systemic Hypersensitivity Associated with Microneedle Therapy for Skin Rejuvenation. JAMA Dermatology. 2014;150(1):68–72. doi:10.1001/jamadermatol.2013.6955

Sowden JM, Byrne JPH, Smith AG, Hiley C, Suazrez V, Wagner B et al. Red Tattoo Reactions: X-ray Microanalysis and Patch-test Studies. British Journal of Dermatology. 1991;124(6):576–80. doi:10.1111/j.1365-2133.1991.tb04954.x

Tan CH, Rasool S, Johnston GA. Contact Dermatitis: Allergic and Irritant. Clinics in Dermatology. 2014;32(1):116–24. doi:https://doi.org/10.1016/j.clindermatol.2013.05.033

Torezan L, Chaves Y, Niwa A, Sanches JAJ, Festa-Neto C, Szeimies RM. A Pilot Split-Face Study Comparing Conventional Methyl Aminolevulinate-Photodynamic Therapy (PDT) with Microneedling-Assisted PDT on Actinically Damaged Skin. Dermatologic Surgery. 2013;39(8):1197–201. doi:10.1111/dsu.12233

Van Damme P, Oosterhuis-Kafeja F, Van der Wielen M, Almagor Y, Sharon O, Levin Y. Safety and Efficacy of a Novel Microneedle Device for Dose Sparing Intradermal Influenza Vaccination in Healthy Adults. Vaccine. 2009;27(3):454–9. doi:https://doi.org/10.1016/j.vaccine.2008.10.077

Vicente-Perez EM, Larrañeta E, McCrudden MTC, Kissenpfennig A, Hegarty S, McCarthy HO et al. Repeat Application of Microneedles Does Not Alter Skin Appearance or Barrier Function and Causes No Measurable Disturbance of Serum Biomarkers of Infection, Inflammation or Immunity in Mice In Vivo. European Journal of Pharmaceutics and Biopharmaceutics. 2017;117:400–7. doi:https://doi.org/10.1016/j.ejpb.2017.04.029

Han Tae Y, Park Kui Y, Ahn Ji Y, Kim Seo W, Jung Hye J, Kim Beom J. Facial Skin Barrier Function Recovery after Microneedle Transdermal Delivery Treatment. Dermatologic Surgery. 2012;38(11):1816–22. doi:10.1111/j.1524-4725.2012.02550.x

Yadav S, Dogra S. A Cutaneous Reaction to Microneedling for Postacne Scarring Caused by Nickel Hypersensitivity. Aesthetic Surgery Journal. 2016;36(4):NP168–NP70. doi:10.1093/asj/sjv229

Index

Note: Page numbers in *italics* indicate figures and **bold** indicate tables in the text.